About Pain

...for those who suffer and their caregivers.

Dr. Rachel B. Aarons LCSW

About Pain:
For those Who Suffer and their Caregivers
Rachel B. Aarons MSW, PhD

Printed in the United States of America

Published by Journey Press
Santa Barbara, California 93101

Library of Congress Control Number: 2015904750

ISBN 978-0-9842327-7-2

Book Design by www.KarrieRoss.com
Cover Photos from istockphoto.com

First Edition
10 9 8 7 6 5 4 3 2 1

Dedication

This book is dedicated to
my younger son, fondly dubbed "Guru Dave,"
and
the amazing men and women who shared their stories,
and
the members of my Unitarian Society Women's
Group who gave their feedback and support during
the writing process.

I am deeply grateful to you all.

Contents

Praise for the Book

Pain is the number one complaint that takes patients to a physician. Today pain management is under attack by state and federal regulators... This book provides an in-depth understanding of the disruptive force of pain on people's lives and useful tools for aiding the emotional fall-out of pain. It puts a human face on those who suffer with chronic pain and is an eloquent plea for humanity and understanding.

~David Bearman MD, Pain Management Specialist.

In her book About Pain, *Dr. Rachel B. Aarons explores the emotional side of pain from a clinical and personal perspective... This book gives us insight into the profound effect pain can have. It is a window into the dark room of the experience of pain.*

~Jeoffrey Benson MD PhD., Board Certified Specialist in Pain Management

This book is a unique guide for helping pain patients reduce and transcend their pain. Skillfully filtered through the wisdom of Dr. Aarons' own clinical and personal experience, About Pain *is an empowering antidote for the helplessness that both pain patients and caregivers feel. Few writers on this complex topic address the hidden gremlins of pain - such elements as self-hatred and guilt - with the personal, courageous and compassionate perspective of Dr. Rachel Aarons.*

~Dr. Jeffrey Friedman, Pain Management Psychologist

An important book for those who suffer with pain and those who treat them. This book is a reminder that we physicians have tools even more important than prescription pad or scalpel: ears to listen to our patients and hearts to respond with care and empathy.

~Dr. Eric Trautwein, Internist.

Foreword

A note to the reader

I'd like to have a conversation with you. I'm talking to you, the reader. I'm going to imagine you listening with rapt attention to what I am about to say.

Thinking of this as a conversation rather than a book I'm starting is definitely more comfortable for me. I can sit down and talk to you but I don't know if I can write a book – at least, not *this* book.

The truth is that this book is exactly the one I have been assiduously avoiding for a very long time. It is not a new idea. It has been a constant possibility beckoning to me for several years, but I have been incapable of sitting down and writing it. I think about it and my thoughts dart off in a different direction. Or they circle repetitively and I end up tired and wanting to go to bed. The notebook I started years ago still sits by my bedside literally gathering dust. So, no book emerges. I have been playing hide-and-seek with this book for a long time.

The subject is *pain*. This is a subject we generally don't dive into with great relish. Pain is something that we want to run away from. Who wants to hear about it? Who want to write about it? Who wants to be with it?

What we will discover is that *not wanting to be with pain* is one of its prominent features. Both as the person who suffers pain and as the one who cares for a person in pain, we are inclined to tiptoe around it, to speak of other things, to pretend it doesn't exist. In either the patient or caregiver role, it's hard to be *in* it – to fully engage with the experience of pain.

Why a book at all? If no one wants to hear it and I don't want to write it, this seems an all-too-obvious question. And I have used it quite successfully as my justification for avoiding this project up till now. I have been telling myself that the subject of this book is just intrinsically too painful. How ridiculous this objection sounds in my head: *a book on pain is painful!* But think about it. It's not a place anyone wants to hang out for hours on end in order to write about it. It's likely not a subject you want to hear about for hours on end either. Perhaps it's not a subject you really enjoy hearing about at all. Yet, nonetheless, you *are* reading this book so there must be something that draws you.

Freud said we move toward pleasure and away from pain. But pain is an incontrovertible aspect of our lives. No matter how we try to resist, it is unavoidable. There is the physical pain of illness and disability. And there is the emotional pain of trauma, depression and anxiety. We may think: "What's the point of focusing on something so unpleasant as pain? The less we say about it the better." As a consequence, the sufferer becomes trapped in isolation; the caregiver in incomprehension. Our pain is magnified in our effort to avoid it.

The implication is that, despite our inclination to be silent on the subject of pain, someone needs to talk about it – in detail, in depth, from all sides. Someone needs to break the taboo and bring it out of the shadows. But, I asked myself, why should that someone be me?

It is a dubious claim to fame that I qualify as a person with extensive experience of pain. I will tell you about my experience – despite my reluctance – because I believe you have a right to know why I am presuming to speak on this topic and why you might benefit by listening to me.

First, I have had my share of physical pain and illness. In 1994, I was diagnosed with fibromyalgia. I suffered with unremitting pain in my body for almost twenty years – in my hands and fingers, arms and shoulders, neck, feet and legs. Some pain took residence in specific parts of my body and some pain was "ambulatory," meaning that it would move around and suddenly attack and torment a part that had been relatively quiet before. My body was so highly sensitized that any touch beyond the lightest and most gentle was painful to me. Being jostled in a crowd, an accidental bump or brush, a vigorous handshake, or an enthusiastic hug would cause me to gasp and recoil uncontrollably. I was one of the virtual "untouchables." As a naturally affectionate and touchy-feely person, this was very difficult for me.

In addition to touch, I was sensitive to light, noise, and cold. If we were traveling west just before sundown with the sun in our eyes, I would be on the verge of a meltdown. I understood all too well why they tortured prisoners with a constant blinding light in their eyes.

Although I had moved to California for the warm dry climate, I was cold all the time. My six layers of clothing were a joke in my Jazzercise class. At home, I would huddle in front of the gas fireplace in my living room so close to the fire that my knees would burn. But I still shivered with the freezing cold that was coming from inside.

Loud noises caused me to start and startle. I stayed away from the noisy party places so popular in this town. Any event involving crowds of people was a challenge for me. The close proximity of bodies, the volume of noise, and the intensity of stimulation left me nervous, dizzy and exhausted. Big gala events were rarely fun for me.

Add to this digestive problems, headaches, and fatigue. I had to spend long stretches of time horizontal because I was too weak or it was too painful for me to be up and around. Understand that I am not, by nature, a lie-around personality. I am, if anything, a compulsive doer. Given the choice, I would rather be busy all the time. My body did not give me a choice.

No matter how much I hated resting, the dizziness and pain would force me to lie down. I never watch TV so looking at the ceiling was not my idea of a good time. I was bored and resentful about the limitations of my condition. I felt trapped in a body that hurt. And that body ruled my life.

Then in 2010, it morphed to a new level. Every day I would come home from work, collapse on the couch, and lie there too weak to feed myself. Trust me, as a "foodie," I had to be totally and completely enervated to be unable to eat! But the worst part was when I started waking up at night in excruciating pain and, at the same time, *paralyzed*. I literally could not move a muscle. I knew there was pain medication on the night table beside me less than six inches away, but I could not reach out to get it. It was a sense of utter helplessness I shall never forget. It took nine months before I received the diagnosis of polymyalgia rheumatica and the medication that would bring me relief.

In 2011, I had arthoscopic knee surgery and my first attack of diverticulitis. In 2013, I had early stage breast cancer with a partial mastectomy and a course of radiation. My oncologist said that a diagnosis of cancer is a traumatic experience in itself, not to mention the medical process that it forces you to go through. Although cancer is never a walk in the park, I was lucky enough to have a relatively easy time since I had a very small tumor and I opted not to do chemotherapy. Instead, I put myself "in training," determined to recover my strength and get into hiking. Exercise would be my Tamoxifen. I trained for nine months for the big hiking trip I took to Sedona in February of 2014. It was a triumph for me.

Maybe I flew too close to the sun or, whatever the reason, in June of that year I began a downward spiral. First, a gnarly GI tract infection; then, a miserable bout of poison oak. But the winner by far was the sixteen days I spent in hospital with a perforated bowel. My stomach blew up like a basketball and the pain came in waves that took my breath away. I was on two Norcos every two hours. If you get the picture, then you can see it was a dreary one.

I went from CT scan to CT scan for over two weeks, praying I would be released from hospital and hearing each time (except for the last,) that I would have to wait another four days. Almost daily my doctor kept reminding me just how sick I was and how I could go "toxic" at any moment. I tried to put that out of my mind.

For the first week, I couldn't eat anything. My doctor ordered milkshakes for me. I've already told you that I am a foodie so the experience of being disinterested in food, much less repelled by it, was entirely new for me.

It is indescribable how *long* sixteen days in hospital can be. Even the nurses commented on how long a stay it was. Yet less than two months later, I was back in hospital for a bowel resection. I am still recovering from that surgery now as I write these words.

I'm not saying that what I went through was worse than anyone else's experience – I know very well this isn't so – just that I know what it is like to be constantly sick and in pain for a number of years. I started to reflect upon the commonalities between different experiences of pain, the themes that those of us who are suffering might want others to know.

Hence the first part of the book will be from the viewpoint of the patient. I believe it needs to be an *inside* point of view. Too often the people who are writing and teaching about pain are coming from the outside perspective. They are not in pain themselves. For example, years ago I took a course on fibromyalgia from a lovely young woman who appeared to be in excellent health. She had memorized the material in the syllabus and spoke from her head with the best of intentions. It rang hollow. She came from outside, not inside, the experience of fibromyalgia. I will speak from the inside of the pain experience. In so doing, I hope to give voice to those in sickness and pain who may never have spoken up for themselves.

At the same time as having a long history of pain, I have an even longer history of being a psychotherapist. As unbelievable as it seems to me, it is actually coming on to *forty* years! I couldn't help musing on the fact that it is the same length of time the Jews wandered in the desert waiting for the Promised Land.

And what is it to be a therapist? It is about working with, being present with, and helping people in pain. Their pain may be physical or emotional or both. Often they go together. An important study casts light on this connection.

The Adverse Childhood Experience (ACE) Study is a major American research project the poses the question of whether, and how, childhood experiences affect adult health decades later. We learn from ACE that there is "a powerful relationship between our emotional experiences as children and our physical and mental health as adults... It documents the conversion of traumatic emotional experiences in childhood into organic disease later in life."[1]

The author goes on to ask: "How does this happen, this reverse alchemy, turning the gold of a newborn infant into the lead of a depressed, diseased adult? The Study makes it clear that time does *not* heal some of the adverse experiences we found so common in the childhoods of a large population of middle-aged, middle class Americans. One does not 'just get over' some things, not even fifty years later."[2]

Dr. Bessel van der Kolk illuminates the connection between trauma and illness when he says:

---

[1] Felitti, Vincent J. M.D. *The Relationship of Adverse Childhood Experience to Adult Health: Turning Gold into Lead,* Kaiser Permanente Medical Care Program, San Diego, California, 2002, p.2.

[2] Weiss J.S. & Wagner S.H. *What explains the negative consequences of adverse childhood experiences on adult health?* American Journal of Preventive Medicine, 1998; 14: 356-360, quoted in Felitti, Vincent, above.

"Under normal circumstances people react to a threat with a temporary increase in their stress hormones. As soon as the threat is over, the hormones dissipate and the body returns to normal. The stress hormones of traumatized people, in contrast, take much longer to return to baseline and spike quickly and disproportionately in response to mildly stressful stimuli. The insidious effects of constantly elevated stress hormones include memory and attention problems, irritability, and sleep disorders. They also contribute to many long-term health issues, depending on which body system is most vulnerable in a particular individual."[3]

If this is so, how can we account for the fact that so many people with health issues do not acknowledge the possibility that they have been traumatized in the past? They may even insist that they had perfectly happy childhoods. Dr. Van der Kolk goes on to explain:

"We now know that there is another possible response to threat, which our scans aren't yet capable of measuring. Some people simply go into denial. Their bodies register the threat, but their conscious minds go on as if nothing has happened. However, even though the mind may learn to ignore the messages from the emotional brain, the alarm signals don't stop. The emotional brain keeps working, and stress hormones keep sending signals to the muscles to tense for action or immobilize in collapse. The physical effects on the organs go unabated until they demand notice when they are expressed as illness. Medications, drugs, and alcohol can also temporarily dull or obliterate unbearable sensations and feelings. But the body continues to keep the score."[4]

Whether conscious of trauma or in denial, clients come to therapy to talk about their pain, to be heard and understood.

[3] Van der Kolk, Bessel M.D. *The Body Keeps the Score: Brain, Mind, and Body in the Healing of Trauma,* Viking by the Penguin Group, New York, 2014, p.46.
[4] *Ibid.*

They come hoping to heal. To the extent that I am effective as a therapist, I need to be able to feel into their experience of pain, to validate and empathize with them. This is a necessary starting point.

But I believe that *more* is required. How many of my new clients report that they have seen previous therapists who, they acknowledged, were supportive and would listen and mirror back what they heard. Without doubt, it was a valuable experience for these clients to be received and resonated with. However, these same clients complained that their head-nodding therapists failed to help them bring about *change*. Despite their therapist's caring concern, they remained stuck in their place of pain. Beyond validation and empathy, we need to offer healing in the form of *reduction or elimination of pain*. We need to find that new perspective or that release from the old destructive pattern that is holding them hostage. We need to help them *rise above* their pain. Keep in mind as you read this book that while Part One will give the unabashedly negative and harshly truthful perspective on pain, Part Three will give the inspiring and more positive perspective.

Part Two will be directed to the caregiver, whether that is a family member, a friend, a licensed professional or an unlicensed companion hired to provide care. I will pay particular attention to the medical practitioners – the nurses and doctors – who staff our hospitals and have such a major impact on the lived experience of patients under their care. The hospital is a world all its own, with a potential to be either a healing or harming place for the vulnerable beings called "patients" trapped inside its walls.

In Part Three of the book, we will address the question: What is to be done about pain? Having walked through the grim reality of pain, we now need to ask: Is there reason for hope? We will explore a variety of possible ways to relieve and manage pain, evaluating whether and how people may find ways to live satisfying lives in spite of their pain conditions.

From the perspective of the book as a whole, it is my hope that my years as a therapist helping people in pain, in combination with my years as a patient in pain myself, will adequately equip me to offer a uniquely personal and at the same time professional point of view. I will share the insights I have gained from both (so to speak) sides of the fence.

PART ONE:

The Inside View

A. Reflections on Pain

1. Pain changes the world you experience.

However you lived before, once you are in pain you can be sure things will be different. There will be things you used to do that you can't do anymore – such as, in my case, playing baseball with my sons or going to a high-impact aerobics class. There will be dreams that need to be revised or abandoned – such as retiring and spending my days digging, weeding and planting in my garden. There will be what can only be regarded as "necessary adjustments."

That is because pain sets *limits.* Sometimes gradually, sometimes suddenly, a wall comes up. You can't move in the same way you did before – the way you probably took for granted when you *could* move like that. Now it hurts. Perhaps a little, perhaps a lot.

If the pain is bad enough, you will feel your body pulling back, contracting, and resisting. Your mind will either be enveloped in it or plotting a way to get out or, at least, to get less pain. A new thought pattern gets launched in your head and develops into an ongoing rumination about how to manage in the world with the least amount of pain.

Depending on the illness, the details will be different. It might be about the distances that need to be traversed from one place to another and whether those distances involve hills or slopes or steps. It may be about the smoothness or hardness of the terrain. Or, almost inevitably, it will be about the weather. Is it cold? Is it damp? Is there rain or snow? Is it windy? Is it hot? Do you have your water bottle? Sunglasses?

Sunscreen? Jacket? Scarf? Mitts? Umbrella? Hat? Cane? And all the necessary medications? How close is the parking? How close are the rest rooms? Is there an elevator? Wheelchair access? Will there be stairs to climb? And which is worse? – climbing up the stairs or climbing down? What is the seating like when you get there? Are the chairs comfortable or will you be squirming in your seat throughout the whole event and then unable to get up when it is done? Will the ambience be frenetic or soothing? A hair shirt or a velvet cloak? Will you disturb other people around you with your grunts and groans? What if you get tired and just want to go home?

There seem to be a million details you can be busy obsessing about. Nowhere in this litany of worries and concerns is the anticipation of pleasure. It is all about minimizing the pain. You are now absorbed in a negative, downright boring, and seemingly endless train of anxious thoughts. And if it is negative and boring to you to think this way, just imagine how negative and boring it must be to listen to. Now you can top it all off with a load of guilt. You are miserable and you are making others miserable too.

But the thoughts are compelling. The walls and limits are real. Different conditions will involve different limitations. But all pain involves limitations of some sort. Perhaps we can aspire to rise above them, but we need to begin by acknowledging their inescapable reality.

No longer is the world experienced as a delightful smorgasbord of possibilities inviting you to step up and enjoy.[5] It has become, instead, a morass of irritating problems to be solved, a jungle of practical challenges to be overcome.

---

[5] We must acknowledge that not everybody lives in a world of delightful possibilities. Many find themselves in a country at war, a neighborhood where violence is an everyday occurrence, a home where alcohol, drugs and domestic violence are rampant, an area of the city where there is a daily threat of assault based on racial discrimination, religious intolerance, sexism and poverty. The level of disruption caused by the advent of pain will be relative to the suffering or stability that preceded it.

Not the least of these challenges may be financial. Being sick can be an expensive proposition. When you are ill, you likely can't work for a period of time – or perhaps indefinitely – so your income stream dries up. At the same time, the medical expenses mount.

Depending on the needs of your particular illness, there may be special devices that are required such as wheel chairs, crutches or hospital beds, and special services such as visiting nurses, around-the-clock caregivers, rehabilitation or physical therapy. Some of this may be covered by insurance – if you have it – and some may not. The time spent dealing with insurance companies can be staggering. It is almost a full time job to fight for coverage and one that is as exhausting as it is time-consuming at a time when your energy is in short supply.

As your finances dwindle, so do the options in your life. You not only are physically incapable of pursuing many things you used to enjoy; you may no longer be able to afford them. How many of the country's homeless population are in this position because of astronomical medical bills? It is frightening to entertain the possibility that at any time illness and pain can suddenly rob you of the style of life that has been yours up to that time.

This rupture of the status quo is not only true for the patient; it is also true for those who share their life. Pain brings about loss and loss brings about pain. They are intertwined. At the extreme, the death of one's loved one creates profound pain and grief as we hear about in Jim's story that follows.

Love, Sex and Death: James B. Horton

The pain I experience is the loss of my wife. We were married for forty-five years.

It is very hard to describe a forty-five year loving relation-ship. At no point did we ever consider leaving each other.

We had our problems but divorce was never an option for us. In this age of divorce, it is little understood what it means to be in such a committed relationship - the security it brings, the sense of being with your best friend, your lover, your soul mate.

I met my wife in 1962 when my father sent me to Antwerp, Belgium to buy diamonds for our family business. She was the office manager of the diamond company I was dealing with. Her legal name was Beatrice Komkommer but her boss called her "Cookie." The name I knew her by was "Kucky", the phonetic spelling of "Cookie." She has always been Kucky to me.

We got married three years after I met her. I invited her to come to New York on her vacation in August. I proposed to her at a party and we got married in Las Vegas on August 27, 1966. We chose to go to Vegas because it seemed a much easier route than arranging a wedding with relatives on two continents. A couple of weeks later, I went to Antwerp and met her family. I remember walking into the room and there were her father, mother, two brothers and a sister, all kissing and hugging one another. They opened their arms to welcome me. Everyone was so loving to each other, as well as to me, that I was in shock. This had never happened in my family. It was so painful to me that I had to leave and stay in a hotel. I never had much contact with them after that.

Kucky loved me unconditionally from the start, but it took me years to accept that. It was a first for me. I was a confused person at that time and I had no understanding of what love was. My parents were married for fifty years but I had no feeling of love between them. In my youth when I asked my father about relationships, what he told me was: "Don't ever love anybody because you'll get hurt." That's all I knew.

Our family was not close. My father was verbally abusive and very difficult to live with. The earliest pain I experienced was living with my father who was an alcoholic. As the first son, I was to inherit the family business, whether I wanted to or not. He himself had wanted to be a doctor but his father sent him to Switzerland for a year to study watch-making. He did not speak French and the Swiss at that time were anti-Semitic. We can only guess what happened there that drove him to become such a hostile, arrogant and crazy person whom I both loved and hated. He changed our name from Horowitz to Horton because he was afraid of our being hurt for being Jewish. I am reminded of Henry Miller's words: "No one hates a Jew more than a Jew." He was rageful and instilled fear in us, especially in my younger brother who was terrified of him. I was forced into the family business and worked for him for twenty years.

Kucky taught me about three things I will never forget and for which I am eternally grateful. They were love, sex and death. As I have said, there was no learning about love in my family. As for sex, it was never discussed. I grew up in the fifties where I was taught there were good girls and bad girls, the ones you married and the ones you didn't. Kucky was an artist and an amazing free spirit. She taught me that sex was wonderful and meant to be enjoyed.

In my family, death was never talked about. My father refused to go to a funeral. He would stay home and have a drink. When my grandfather died, he had someone else tell me. When my grandmother died, she was never spoken of again. Then, when my father died, my mother never spoke about him again. Death was treated as a family secret in our family.

For Kucky, death was a natural occurrence. She believed that after death there was nothing. Nothing to fear. No pain. Except the pain of the one left behind.

That pain is indescribable. Kucky had lung cancer as well as Parkinson's and what she went through was terrible. Just after she got lung cancer, she wrote this note to me:

> "Thinking back to those days, even with the difficulties I am having now with my health, my spirit is so much more at peace now. Getting sober and staying sober

was the hardest road I had to travel in my life. After that I feel that I can handle everything that comes at me, with a little help from the universe of course. I feel that I had a blessed life and I will fight hard of course to regain my health. But if this is the beginning of the end, I hope I can accept that graciously too.

I am grateful that I have witnessed and am still witnessing the miracle of our son Jamie's passionate fatherhood.

Love you. Kucky"

She was a person of courage, perhaps even more so than me. The pain of watching her suffer was overwhelming and almost unbearable for me.

It is almost four years since Kucky died. Part of me can't believe it. I know it is true but I still can't believe she's not there. She was the person I had dinner with every night. She was at my side for forty-five years. I didn't know how to cope without her. Being alone was unendurable. I didn't think I could survive.

The worst part was trying to live alone after all those years of living in partnership. The first two months, I tried to date every single woman I met, thinking I had to find a partner. I actually asked two different women to live with me. I kept avoiding being in the condo because Kucky wasn't there. I ran around looking like the happiest person on earth. I was in denial.

Therapy and my hospice counseling have helped me. I am beginning to think that maybe I *can* live alone. After her death, the best question I was asked was: How are you going to fill up your life now? My answer is: I have a lot of friends; I do yoga, walk, hike, swim, read and I love seeing my grandchildren. I feel better than I have ever felt in my life. Kucky's spirit is in me and I still love her. Thanks to Kucky, I know what it is to love.

* * *

Along with the limits and walls, go the *losses*. It is not so easy letting go of those hopes and dreams you have cherished. At the same time as the world becomes weighted down with negativity, it shrinks in options. Many of the enticing possibilities disappear. Either physically or emotionally, they simply are not possibilities anymore.

At bottom, pain constitutes an assault on your freedom of choice in the world. Others get to do so many exciting things while you are walled in by can'ts. Even if your mind is willing, your body may not be. Imagine the frustration of being trapped in a body that is limping, creaky and hurting. You may feel old long before your time. As the world shrinks and sours, it will inevitably affect the person you are.

2. Pain changes the person you are.

People in pain get cranky and cantankerous. Surely it is not so difficult to understand why.

Just tolerating the pain itself takes effort and a force of will. It's an effort to keep your spirits up and this effort is tiring. Your tone of voice may register strain and this may be perceived as anger and criticism. At the same time, when you are tired and hurting, you get irritated more easily and therefore are perceived as irritable. Sometimes that perception is correct. You really are angry at the situation you are in.

Add to this the characteristic feelings that assault the person in chronic or acute pain. You will likely be *depressed*. There is less pleasure in the present; there is less to look forward to in the future. You may be worrying about whether this is a temporary or permanent state. Or you may see it not only as not getting better but as inevitably getting worse.

When one of my clients with cancer had back surgery, the surgeon assured her in advance that she would feel no more pain in her back. He was right. The surgery paralyzed her and she could feel nothing from her neck down. Confined to a wheel chair and unable to care for herself, this independent woman was deeply depressed. It seems to me that she had every right to be.

Being sick and in pain radically diminishes your quality of life. It can be deeply disappointing and crushingly sad. What came home to me from my first surgery (the cancer one) was the conviction that if you want something, *go after it!* Don't wait for the right time – when you finally have enough money or time or the kids are grown or the job is done or the mortgage is paid. "Do it now!" became my motto. Because the so-called "right" time may never come.

Overnight your life may be drastically altered. You may be running to doctors' appointments and procedures and labs so often that it feels like you just added a second full-time job. Or, as in the case of my second surgery, you may go to the hospital expecting to pick up some medication and find yourself instead being immediately admitted to intensive care. This could be the beginning of a drama that will play out for the next several weeks, months or, it could be, years.

Both my surgeons and my oncologist maintain that depression is a predictable and entirely "normal" result of major surgery, even if the surgery is successful. Not only is the process physically taxing and inescapably painful. It also brings you face to face with your fundamental vulnerability.

If you ever imagined you were in control of your life, this experience flies in the face of that presumption, exposing the arrogance that lies behind it. Rarely do people consciously and purposely make themselves sick. Most of the time it just "happens" to them. It is something that is not under their conscious control. How unnerving to have your life turned upside down without any choice on your part. How devastating to be caught up in a nightmare that has become your life while you were busy planning other things.

Hence, powerlessness, helplessness, and lack of control are themes that play out in the world of illness and pain. We are harshly reminded of the frailty of our bodies, the fact that we are fundamentally physical beings subject to the vicissitudes of pain, disease and death.

3. Pain generates anger.

This awareness generates a protest. You may want to rail against your fate and upbraid the powers-that-be for creating such an unjust world. You may want to yell at God, the creator of this mess, for allowing this to happen. You may even give up on the possibility that a God exists at all.

Alternatively, you may settle for second best and satisfy your rage by yelling at the caregiver who is right there beside your bed.

People in pain are likely to be *angry*. We may feel like we want to birch and complain all the time. "Why me? It isn't fair! I don't deserve to suffer this way!" You may want to go into excruciating detail about everything that is happening to you. "This throbs; that aches; this burns; that pounds." And truth be told, you may be jealous and resentful that it is happening to you and not somebody else.

Some people give themselves permission to express their anger at anyone or everyone who is around. A person like this on a hospital ward gets known pretty quickly. This is no accident. This sort of person *wants* to make their presence known. It must feel better on some level to make your protest heard and not just take it quietly "lying down."

Most of us are more inhibited. We try to hold back and contain our anger. Perhaps we have moral compunctions against being offensive to others. Perhaps we are sheltering others from knowing about our pain. Or perhaps we are exercising self-protection in not wanting to alienate the people we depend on in our support system. We don't want them to turn against us and walk away.

Nonetheless, our anger may leak out in a tone of impatience and irritation. We may sound critical and ungrateful. Since pleasure has receded from our ongoing experience, it is hard to be pleased with anything in our life. Then we hear ourselves being snippy and crotchety. At best it will be disconcerting and, at worst, deplorable to become aware of how easily we can slip into victim mode during painful episodes of this sort. Again, guilt and shame rear their ugly heads and we feel bad about ourselves for our grumpiness.

So we put on a brave front and keep up appearances. We know that pain is a "downer" and we don't want to bring others down. We put on an act and pretend we're feeling better than we are. On the surface, everything is pleasant and positive. Our inner suffering selves are hidden from view.

One hard day after a long time of being ill and pretending, I wrote this rant about the toll it takes to keep up this hypocrisy. It speaks of Santa Barbara where I live but you can apply it to other places too.

> *You gotta smile! Say you're fine. It's fine. Everything is fine, fine, fine. Take a positive attitude. No one wants to hear your troubles. No one cares about your pain. Don't be a drag to be around. Smile and lighten their day.*

> *You need to be fun! It's all about fun. What else is there? What else could there be? The Santa Barbara Sing-song Society is all about fun, fun, fun. Don't get all serious. Don't whine and complain. Forget that reality is a conjunction of opposites – the dark and the light, the good and the bad, the blessings and tragedies. We only*

*want to see/hear/think about the lightness and bright-
ness. The healthy and the strong.*

*Get the troubled, homeless, sick and crazy people off the
streets so we don't need to face them. Don't let their pain
blemish your day - your visit to the spa, your pedicure,
your cocktails on the patio. Begone with your dirt and
suffering, your messed up ugly bodies, your hopelessly
disturbed minds. Keep the world antiseptic. Smile and it's
all okay.*

4. Pain fragments the self.

We can see that a split has developed between the way we act
on the surface and the way we feel inside. This distance
between appearance and reality creates a sense of isolation
and loneliness. We can't let others into our inner experience.
Who we really are underneath is invisible. As a result, people in
pain are likely to feel *alone and disconnected.*

Being in pain is intrinsically lonely. It is a solitary
experience that nobody can share. No one else can feel what
you feel. No one else can be inside your body and know
what you are going through. Even if you wanted to communicate your inner experience, it is difficult to find the language
to do so. Pain is in the realm of the unutterable.

As philosopher Elaine Scarry says: "Physical pain does not
simply resist language but actively destroys it, bringing about an
immediate reversion to a state anterior to language, to the
sounds and cries a human being makes before language is
learned...[I]ts resistance to language is not simply one of its
incidental or accidental attributes but is essential to what it is."[6]

---

[6] Scarry, Elaine: *The Body in Pain: The Making and Unmaking of the World*, Oxford
University Press, New York, 1985, pp. 4 - 5.

We feebly turn to metaphors and analogies. "It's pounding like a hammer; it's stinging like a bee; it's dragging me down like an ocean wave; it's burning like a firey blaze." The hammers, bees, waves and fires point toward an experience that can't be directly expressed in words. Perhaps groans and moans and screams come closer. It's rather like being locked in prison. Others can come to visit but, unlike you, they get to leave. They don't have to live in your cell.

Nor would they want to. Being sick and in pain is a blow to our sense of self. It is not an appealing prospect. One of the reasons I avoided writing this book was, I admit, a horror of being seen as a person in pain. It brings up *shame*. When you go through the world wincing and struggling to move, you feel different from other, healthy, people. And with that difference comes a sense of being *less than* or *not as good*.

The fact is, there is a stigma attached to being in pain that makes it shameful. It is as if there is an unspoken assumption that if you had it "together," you wouldn't be in pain. You would be in a sound body, healthy and vibrant. So there must be something wrong with you psychologically if you are going through so much bodily pain.

Now, you not only have to put up with the pain in your body. You also have to feel bad about yourself for having it. Somehow – although you likely have *no* idea how – you are to blame for your suffering. It is a sign to the world that you are damaged on some deep internal level. And this damage is being broadcast to the world.

So you pull back from making contact with people and exposing your imperfections. Although you want and need connection, there is a powerful tendency to isolate. You feel judged by others and you judge yourself. You are embarrassed to be seen in the world. You retreat and isolate.

5. Pain transforms your experience of time.

If you are sick for a long time, your own movement toward isolation may be simultaneously accelerated by friends and family. Their visits may diminish. Their cards and calls and emails may cease to appear. People go back to their lives and time passes. For a person in pain, it can be an eternity from morning to night whereas weeks fly by for healthy people. Their perception of time is radically different. A friend thought she had just been there to see me. She was shocked to discover it had, in fact, been three weeks earlier.

Pain changes the experience of time in two complementary directions. At once stretching out and being endlessly expansive, it feels like it will never end. At the same time, it contracts and concentrates exclusively on the fierceness of the moment. It is like a bottomless pit. Intense pain feels unbearable and, in that moment, it is all that exists. Pain thus conveys the paradox of the eternal now that lasts forever. In relation to pain, it is a terrifying prospect to behold.

Hopelessness is thus intrinsic to the lived experience of intense pain. We may be reassured by others that it will stop but, in the moment, it is impossible to believe. Our subjective bodily experience belies whatever the mind has to say. Despair may be virtually insurmountable.

There are precious fibers that bind us to life. These are, according to Buddhism, the attachments that cause us to suffer. They are also what make life meaningful. Pain and illness gnaw at these fibers like the mouse in the Zen parable gnawing at the rope that holds a man perilously suspended over a cliff. We become more and more detached and disconnected as life goes on without us. We feel excluded, even forgotten. And the prison cell that remains our lot in life cannot begin to make up for the growing loss of the world.

Pain may systematically attack everything we are attached to. In my case, it was first travel, then gardening, then taking long walks and going out with friends. When I finally tried to adjust to a solitary and sedentary life by beginning to work on a book, my body launched a new attack on me. Frozen shoulders, carpel tunnel, swollen hands. If I couldn't work on the computer, how was I to write? I wondered what message my body in its mercilessness was sending me.

In the middle of the night after I had groped my way to the pain medication and it was finally beginning to cut in, everything was quiet and I felt calm. The message was crystal clear. My body was putting me through disengagement training. I was learning to detach, Buddhist style.

6. Pain fosters self-hatred.

At the same time as you are turning away from others, you will also be turning away from yourself. The experience of being in unceasing and intolerable pain feels very much like being tormented. Who is the tormenter that treats you this way? It is *your own body*. The despot who subjects you to this torture is an intimate part of yourself.

Pain is like a prison – in more ways than one. It never feels chosen. It is almost always forced upon you against your will. You are compelled to be locked inside it indefinitely. You aren't free to check out of your body, although you can make efforts to dissociate. To the degree that it is possible, not feeling your body's pain is often the best way to manage it.

Dissociation is a method of removing oneself from that which is intolerable. It may start early in life as a response to abuse – emotional, physical or sexual abuse – and become a spontaneous and habitual reaction. When we are physically unable to run away from a situation, our only escape route may be in our minds. When the perpetrator of the intolerable is not outside but inside us, we may try to stop feeling connected to our body. We put our awareness somewhere else.

It is interesting to note that those who have been abused in childhood may have perfected this defense mechanism. Since, according to the ACE study, these are the children more likely to have disease, addiction and chronic pain as adults later in life, they have been well prepared by their abuse to utilize this defense to cope with their pain.

Of course, we try a multitude of other ways. Sometimes they are helpful and sometimes not.

It's such a shock when you think you are doing better and then all of a sudden you're not. I rested, I drank my obnoxious green drink, I ate everything I should. I only spent fifteen minutes on the computer and I passed up my Jazzercise class. I took a pain killer and went to bed early. I woke up racked with pain and paralyzed. I was in the suit of armor again.

I wanted to protest: "But I did everything right! I did everything I was supposed to! I was a very good girl so why am I being punished? Why am I being dropped into the pain pit again?"

The response from my body was like a sharp rap on the knuckles harshly reminding me that I am not the one in control. It doesn't need to be fair. It can be completely capricious and without reason. My body can be cruel and malicious. It owed no explanation to me.

Now we are genuinely turned against ourselves. My body versus me. This is almost certainly the deepest form of betrayal when it is your own body that is the enemy. How can we come to terms with being locked inside a body that abuses us in this way?

It may seem that we are condemned, without reprieve, to live in a body that hates us. And we may come to hate our body in return. Is there a way out then? Do we humbly submit to our fate or decide to take action?

7. Pain forces us to confront life and death.

Suspended over the cliff, staring into the abyss, we are face to face with one of the wrenching and highly controversial issues of our time: it is the issue of *suicide*.

It is a legal, moral and religious issue. Our prevailing cultural belief is that suicide is wrong and is to be resisted, at all cost. Only three states in the United States of America (Oregon, Washington and Vermont) have legalized assisted suicide. The rest of the country retains legislation that is opposed. Yet Wikipedia reports that: "According to several studies, more than half of the oncologists polled have received requests from a patient wanting to end their life."[7] What this means is that if you are suffering so much that life has become unbearable and you turn to your physician for help, it is *illegal* for him or her to help you. To do so would be to run against the Hippocratic Oath that binds a physician to protect and sustain life. The assumption underlying this oath is that sustaining life is always in the best interest of the patient. But is this always true?

Similarly, as therapists, we have a mandate to report a client at risk of suicide so that authorities can step in to prevent the client from acting. It is argued that the client may act out of a state of despair that is temporary and would pass if a sufficient opportunity were provided. In support of this position, there is evidence that people who attempt suicide and fail are often grateful later that they were unsuccessful.

---

[7] http://en.wikipedia.org/wiki/Assisted_suicide

Some religions condemn suicide and insist that people who kill themselves will be sent to hell or, at least, prohibited from being welcomed into heaven. Some religions extol as martyrs monks who immolate themselves or suicide bombers who blow themselves up for political causes. What is regarded as sinful by some can be revered as saintly by others.

I do not intend to tackle the thorny legal, moral and religious issue of suicide here. I have a much smaller lens. I just want to address the issue from the specific vantage point of the person in intense pain.[8]

When a person experiences pain that is extreme and overwhelming for a long time – long enough for us to have had numerous episodes of finding it unbearable, I think it fair to conjecture that our thoughts may turn to wanting it to end. It is like being asked to live the unliveable. Without doubt, intense pain can take us to the brink. Further, if we are also convinced that our condition is untreatable and that this level of pain will be our inescapable companion every moment in the future, we may find ourselves reluctant – or, at least, conflicted – about going forward with a life that is dominated by intolerable pain.

On the last point, it may be objected that there is always the possibility of something new and different impacting the situation – a new discovery or some unforeseeable shift. Actually, this was true in my case.

After nine months of trying every remedy offered and finding none helpful in addressing the agony of my condition, I decided as a last resort to see a new rheumatologist. Within twenty-four hours, he had diagnosed my condition and given me medication that virtually obliterated the pain.

---

[8] I would imagine that there is an equivalent issue for people in states of disability that may make carrying on with life as unendurable as those who are suffering intense pain. Sometimes, tragically, they have to deal with both disability and pain.

It turned out that for the previous nine months, I had suffered due to the incompetence of my earlier physician who failed to recognize a disease (polymyalgia rheumatica) well known within his area of specialization, and one that was treated by a medication (Prednisone) that had been equally well known for many years. What had seemed absolutely irremediable during those nine months of torture completely reversed within a day. This was what happened to me. It could happen to anyone. You just don't know.

Does that mean that we should never give up regardless of how hopeless our situation may appear to be? I'm not sure we can dictate an answer – pro or con – to this question. I think it may only be answerable by each patient for him or herself.[9] Do you think we have the right to override another individual's right to be the author of his or her own life and death? Would you want to surrender that right yourself? Would you want to let the person you care about suffer indefinitely – even if that person is yourself?

Living with and genuinely struggling with the possibility of ending your life ushers you into an extraordinarily strange state of consciousness. It is as if you are moving among people but are no longer one of them. I believe this is how *alienation* feels. What is going on inside separates you irrevocably from the people around you. On the surface you are acting as if everything is unchanged, but the truth is that everything is profoundly different. You are living with death at your side.

On some level, we all know that each and every one of us will die, but most of us do not focus on it. We push the knowledge out of our everyday consciousness and act *as if* it were not so.

---

[9] The issue of competency is sure to arise in the discussion at this point. I will not go into that issue here except to comment that whenever we sanction outside agents to make decisions about a person's life, there is always potential for that power to be abused.

Most of us live like water beetles – skimming along the surface of life – more or less mindlessly going through the motions in a dazed repetitive way. But pain can pierce through this veil of mindlessness. It can be a strident wake-up call. You are forcibly ejected out of the normalcy of your ordinary life and flung into a radically different world, a world that none of us would choose for ourselves – a world of suffering.

And that world is very personal. It is not a vague abstraction like "human suffering." The suffering is *mine*. It is not human mortality in general but *my death* that is on the line.

There is a remarkably strong survival force inside each of us that clings to life tenaciously. It is difficult to grasp the possibility that we would – actually and seriously – choose to let it go. It is hard to wrap our heads around the idea of not existing – to imagine the world without ourselves being in it. One part may be imagining not breathing while another part is gasping for air. It can be no less than an epic battle that must be waged in the struggle between life and death.

Sitting in the force-field of this choice is surprisingly clarifying. It will likely create a shake-down of your familiar world. What is worth living for and what really doesn't matter? Confronting this question forces you to reevaluate your life. Some things simply lose importance when time is short. As a striking example, it seemed pointless and frankly absurd to be struggling to lose weight. Moreover, what was the point of worrying about money, I thought, although I had done so almost my whole life? There wouldn't be much time to spend it anyway so I might as well be spending it on what I liked. In fact, one might ask, why waste time doing *anything* you didn't like? Or being with people who were difficult to take? As a therapist, I began to have less patience. Patience implies an abundance of time. I felt an inclination to "cut to the chase" and be more blatantly honest in my feedback to clients. I was less willing to skirt around the truth.

Ironically, facing death can bring an exhilarating, albeit frightening, sense of freedom. This is not the outer freedom to pursue activities but the inner freedom to be ourselves. If you use awareness of death as a wake-up call, it pierces through the layers of should's and have-to's boring its way down to what really matters. We get a truer, clearer picture of who we are.

Perhaps when we are released from the overriding concern for social obligations and protocol, we also start seeing others more clearly. By analogy, it is as if we were alcoholics who sobered up and were able to see our drinking buddies through fresh eyes. "They think they're funny but they're being obnoxious." "They think they are running away from their issues but there they are spilling out all around them." You see the games – at least those in which you are not co-opted. Being alienated – that is, being among them but not of them – gives you a unique perspective. With death at our side, we are closer to truth.

It's a heady, almost mind-altering state. But not an easy one.

In the end, facing death is like a gritty values clarification exercise. You find out what really matters to you after, as the saying goes, "all is said and done." However, the difference is: this is no exercise. This is the real thing.

B. Voices of Pain

Physical pain has no voice, but when it at last finds a voice, it begins to tell a story.[10]

In this section, we will hear from other people besides myself who have experience with severe pain. They include lay people and professionals, males and females, people of different ages and temperaments, people with a variety of different medical conditions that they have managed in the past or manage still.

They have agreed to write about their personal experiences so that you can learn from them. Perhaps they will give you some insight into what you are going through in your own painful illness and offer validation from real people who suffer as you do. Perhaps they have a message to give to the professionals who treat illnesses like theirs and may discover in what ways they succeed – and fail – in their attempts to help. Or perhaps they can offer a meaningful perspective to those with loved ones who are suffering but unable to communicate their needs.

Whatever the impact of their writing, I cannot emphasize enough the immense gratitude I feel that they have decided to share their truth with us. I know all too well just how difficult it is to do what they are doing and the courage and generosity of spirit it requires. To give voice to what is often lived in silence and speak about the unspeakable is no mean feat.

* * *

---

[10]Scarry, Elaine: *The Body in Pain: The Making and Unmaking of the World*, p. 3.

Eleven Patient Stories

1. Pain Brings Me Home
   Back Surgery: Marilyn J. Owen

2. My Journey With My "Frenemy"
   Back Pain and Other Problems: Michael Vogel

3. Pain Stops Your Life
   Bulging Discs: Pat G.

4. Thirty Years a Slave to Pain
   Workplace Accident: Rick

5. The Way Out is the Way In
   Sports Accident: Wendy Allen

6. A Third of My Life
   Migraine Headaches: Pete

7. Just Breathe
   Leucemia: Nancy Monnie

8. Elevator Ride with Pain
   I. Open Heart Surgeries: Otis
   II.Cancer: Otis

9. The Body Remembers
   Ectopic Pregnancy: Louise Currey

10. Not an Easy Life
    Brain Tumor: Justin

11. Pain By Design
    Shattered Ankle: David Eagle

1. Pain Brings Me Home

Back Surgery: Marilyn J. Owen, MA, LMFT

It seems the only thing that slows me down enough to actually feel my body—the most intimate home I will ever have—is physical pain.

Pain brings me home. This is what comes to mind as I drop to the floor, gingerly and with little grace, to stretch the stiffness and pain from my aching body. Indelicate groans and colorful language fall out of my mouth. I've been pushing myself too hard today, both on my feet and sitting at the computer. Oh, and yesterday, too. And the day before. It doesn't take much to go past my limit these days, and yet I continue to do so as I always have. It seems the only thing that slows me down enough to actually feel my body—the most intimate home I will ever have—is physical pain.

A rueful smile comes next. I breathe into my lower back, bunched up in a spasm of holding on, and encourage her to let go. I imagine her magically melting into the floor. She does not do my bidding. Why should she? I have been ignoring her for weeks. From the book, *Coming Home to Myself*, Marion Woodman's admonition surfaces: "A body whose wisdom has never been honored does not easily trust. An animal with a crazy trainer learns crazy habits, runs wild." It is fitting for me to remember that a lifetime of crazy habits eventually led me to major spine surgery two years ago, and a long recovery. I have learned a little since then, slowly but slowly.

It is now understood that there is an intimate connection between the body and the psyche. In fact, it might be more accurate to say there is no connection, because there is no separation. Physical symptom is as rooted in our psychology as our psychology arises from our physical being. This became clear to me as I worked through many years of psychotherapy and then found myself in physical therapy in an attempt to avoid surgery. In therapy, I had come to understand that I had rather poor boundaries and was overly flexible in my desire to meet the needs of others. It took a long time to learn to say "no", express anger when necessary, set limits, and take care of myself before taking care of everyone else. There was a period of acknowledging and grieving my experience of not having the support I needed to be secure in the world, and a period when I had to take responsibility for how I routinely failed to support myself emotionally, physically, and spiritually.

When my physical therapist described what she saw in my spine, she said I was "extremely flexible," but didn't have enough strength in my core to keep the backbone supported. Adding to the problem, I had a hairline fracture in the lower spine, which made it even more unstable, and slight curvature in the mid-back. These were fundamental structural problems I was born with, but too little exercise and too much weight had contributed to an untenable situation that I could not fix on my own.

It was a short leap to see how my body had manifested my psychic situation. Indeed, I needed to have more backbone (personal boundaries) if I wanted to walk (move forward in life) without increasing pain. Eventually, the surgeon did his part by implanting titanium supports and fusing discs, and I did my part by making radical changes in my professional and personal life. Both of these efforts led to a dramatic reduction in pain on all fronts.

And yet, here I am on the floor. Hurting. I turn again to Woodman, whose life work was around growing a deep capacity for compassion toward the body. She tells us: "Often we listen to a cat with more precision than we listen to our body. We cherish the cat. It purrs. Our body may have to release a scream, a symptom, to be heard by us at all. Too often our soul can find no other way to be heard" (1998, p. 47). What is my body-soul telling me today? She is telling me I need to get to the pool for strengthening and stretching, if I expect to sit for eight or more hours a day seeing clients or attending to a computer screen. She is telling me to be present and listen *right now*.

Ok, I'm listening. I'm breathing into the pain instead of medicating or distracting myself with a computer screen. I'm giving it voice instead of contracting into quiet endurance. I'm moving to internal music instead of freezing into unconscious postures of concentration. Amazingly, I feel her melting into the floor just a bit, as if to say, "NOW, I can relax a little. Now that you are *with* me."

My final thoughts here are gratitude for the pain I have experienced because of the wisdom that came after. Woodman teaches us: "This is your body, your greatest gift, pregnant with wisdom you do not hear, grief you thought was forgotten, and joy you have never known" (p. 49). Indeed, wisdom seems to only come from suffering. The measure of joy we can hold is equal to the measure of grief we can tolerate. I'm grateful for pain as my body's way of reminding me to reorient my awareness toward her – to return home.

*   *   *

Reference:

Woodman, W. & Mellick, J., *Coming home to myself: Daily reflections for a woman's body and soul.* Conari Press: Berkeley, California, 1998.

2. My Journey With My "Frenemy"

Back Pain and Other Problems: Michael Vogel

Pain is both my friend and my enemy. In July of 1993, I was deployed with my combat squadron in the desert of Nevada, nearing the end of three months of rigorous flying as we got ready to deploy to the Persian Gulf. I was a carrier-based attack pilot, with eight years of active duty in the U.S. Navy and I was nearing a critical transition point from junior officer to the pipeline of command. I had not seen much of my family over those eight years due to deployments and training, but I was dedicated to my career. I loved being paid to fly tactical jets aboard aircraft carriers at sea. There was nothing like the thrill of taking off from an aircraft carrier at sea, flying a mission, and then returning to the deck, even in bad weather. It was a dream job and I was good at it.

Over a period of three weeks, I began to have a nagging pain in my left leg and buttocks region. Reluctantly I went to see our squadron flight surgeon to get it checked out. He examined me and found me fit to return to duty saying: "You just have a pulled muscle. Take it easy and cut back on your exercise until it heals."

I returned to flying, but as the endless missions wore on, I began to struggle getting in and out of the cockpit. After one long night flight, I woke up the next morning unable to move. No matter what position I tried, I could not find comfort from the searing pain down my left leg and in my lower back. I hobbled to the base medical clinic and met with my flight surgeon again. This time he put me on muscle relaxants and pain killers but the pain got progressively worse as each day elapsed. After a week of this torture, I was finally medivac'd to the Naval Hospital in San Diego, where surgery was performed on my L4-L5 disc. I recovered quickly, thinking the worst was over and I would soon return to active duty.

My squadron deployed without me and I continued to progress in my rehabilitation, though some of the pain remained. After rehab, I returned to partial duty but the pain steadily returned to haunt me. I went back to the surgeon and he simply dismissed it as phantom pain. But I knew that something was wrong.

I spent the next nine months persevering through the pain with minimal pain medication and continuing to follow the regimen of physical exercise. All of this enormous effort should have helped me return to full active duty but my efforts were not paying off. After much complaining, my surgeon reluctantly agreed to another CT scan. Just as I had predicted and much to the chagrin of my surgeon, the disc had failed again. I underwent yet another surgery, my second in a nine month period, but this one turned out to be a career ender. A week after my surgery and just about the same time I arrived home, I received a letter from the Naval Medical Aeronautics Command stating that I was permanently barred from further flight duties. I was devastated by this news and I sunk into a severe depression. My dream of a career in the military had abruptly ended.

> Disabled and depressed, I was discharged from Naval Service with very little compensation and thrown into impoverishment with a wife and disabled child to support.

The combination of this financial burden coupled with the psychological distress, an enormous amount of residual pain, and the beginning of an autoimmune disease naturally exacerbated the pain symptoms. Pain had become my enemy and my master. I did not know where to turn and what to do with this beast. The U.S. military medical system is well equipped to keep its service members strong and healthy, but rather poorly equipped to treat those who are suffering from permanently disabling conditions. On the heels of all this trauma, I began to have some gastric issues that would eventually be diagnosed as Crohn's-Enterocolitis, a new addition to my pain constellation.

In an ironic twist of fate that fully explained my continued chronic pain, I found out that the two failed surgeries were performed by an unqualified Navy neurosurgeon, who had slipped through the cracks of the government bureaucracy. After a very expensive fight for compensation for the series of medical blunders I had experienced, I was finally afforded some comfort from my ordeal by the civilian medical system, but that is not what this story is about. What it is about is how I came back to a somewhat active and fulfilling career as a psychologist.

You may ask why I use the word *frenemy* to characterize my pain. I see it as a combination of friend and enemy. Pain is our body's way of telling us that something is wrong with the system as a result of physical trauma. For most people, pain syndrome will cause them to reevaluate their current course of action to protect the body (and sometimes the mind) from further injury. This is why I consider it my friend but, like most friends, it has its shadow side.

Just as with an antisocial friend, one has to take great care not to upset the body-mind system with unrealistic expectations or demands.

My current physical body is no different. I have spent years listening and having serious conversations with my body. This does not mean that I ask nothing of it and treat it with kid gloves. I have become very adept at knowing what my physical limitations and boundaries have become. This involves a never ending heart-to-heart conversation and the conditions change from day to day. One day I might go out until late in the evening, but that is accomplished as a result of prior planning, exercise and rest. Most days I keep a very rigid schedule of meditation, relaxation techniques and exercise, so that I can spend time engaging in loving relationships that provide a sense of satisfaction, as well as distraction, from my *frenemy*.

Few disabilities come in an isolated package of one single diagnosis. As with most patients, I have multiple diagnoses: degenerative disc disease at multiple spinal levels, rheumatoid arthritis, Crohn's disease, migraines, mood disorder, sleep disorder, idiopathic neuropathy and chronic pain. All of these diagnoses come with medications, some with uncomfortable side effects. I have come to accept the bad with the good, working closely with my physicians to find the best overall result. I have accepted the fact that I will never be a perfect specimen, a key ingredient in finding self-acceptance. I have learned to imagine myself in a new light, not as a reject, but as someone with a great deal of life experience that can be translated into knowledge. What I have learned about myself through psychology and medicine has developed into a unique knowledge of myself that I can now use to help others find their own meaning within the imaginal realm of pain.

Pain syndrome in any form—physical or psychological—is and can be excruciating, but it does not have to rule your life. Instead you can learn to use it just like any positive attribute or talent you may have in your personality or physicality. For me, my injuries and pain have led me to embrace a more important aspect of my life—relationship. I believe my psyche was asking me to slow down and take stock with regard to my future plan. I had to shed the self-indulgent idea of a career as a Naval Aviator and ultimately as an Admiral in the U.S. Navy. I have found something much more important in life—my family relationships.

I came from a family of poor attachment and I realized that I was following in the same pattern with my own family. I rarely saw my wife and child because I thought my career was the most important priority in my life. Fate stepped in and changed all that following my injury. Admittedly, the nearly sixteen-year process of stabilizing the initial injury and subsequent autoimmune diseases were no picnic. I certainly resisted the process at every level. I was convinced that I did not need anyone to tell me what to do with my body. I was my own man, capable of recovering on my own. But I was wrong!

I needed others to help me find the tools to heal and take care of the new body I was assigned. The physical and psychological tools I was taught over the years actually brought me to a life of fulfillment in both work and relationship. Don't get me wrong. Every day is a new day and a new challenge. Every day can be a bit of a struggle as it brings with it a new set of aches, pains and ever shifting moods, but I am better equipped to manage them. When one becomes more aware of what constitutes a "bad" day and the new definition of a "good" day, one can find joy in the present moment experiences of relationship. It is relationship that brings me to greater gratitude for my current condition and, without relationship, I could never know the higher levels of happiness in my life. This *frenemy* gives me insight and meaning in my life. Learning who I am in our work-oriented society and finding resources to compensate for the added burden of a disability is difficult. It takes perseverance but never lose hope. There is help out there; just keep asking.

* * *

Michael A. Vogel is a retired Navy Lieutenant with ten years active service. He is currently a nearly licensed Marriage and Family Therapist. He is a graduate of California State University, Long Beach with a Bachelors of Science, and Pacifica Graduate Institute where he has completed his Master's of Arts in Counseling Psychology and is currently finishing his Doctorate of Philosophy in Depth Psychology with an emphasis in psychotherapy. He resides in Santa Barbara California with his wife Jennifer and their three children.

3. Pain Stops Your Life

Bulging Discs: Pat G.

My experience with pain came in the fall of 2012 from three herniated disks in my spine. It started out as just a pain in my neck which the doctor at Urgent Care treated with Prednisone. It seemed to work a little in the beginning, but the pain in my neck progressively got worse and I had tingling and numbing in my right forefinger.

Various doctors tried me on at least seven different medications, some of which did nothing at all, and some made me very sick. I was scheduled for an MRI but was in such excruciating pain that I could not lie on the table to have the procedure. I was given more medication and sent back to have the procedure a second time.

I do not remember the procedure at all, as I was in such a daze, but it showed the bulging disks and I was referred to a neurosurgeon. Surprisingly, the neurosurgeon wasn't eager to do surgery and he gave me the options of trying medication first, steroid injections second, and surgery as a last resort. Surgery was not something I was interested in.

One of the bulging disks was pressing on a nerve and the pain shooting down my right arm was almost unbearable. I had never experienced such pain in my life; never having given birth, or even been in the hospital for anything serious. There was nothing that I could do to stop the pain – no body position helped, it was almost impossible to sleep, and I couldn't ride in a car because even the slightest movement would send horrendous pain shooting into my arm.

I was unable to work for over a month and I felt very guilty about that. Days would go by and I would have done nothing but lay in bed or on the couch. The pain was so overwhelming that I wasn't able to read or watch TV. Most nights I would sob myself to sleep. I would call the neurosurgeon begging him to find another medication I could try.

Luckily, my mother lives not far from me. She was such a help doing everything around the house, preparing meals, grocery shopping, taking me to doctor appointments, etc. I could not have done any of those things myself. It was a struggle just to take a shower each day.

In conjunction with the medications, I had a total of three steroid injections. I'm not sure if it was the last medication we tried (Prednisolone Dose Pack) that worked, or the steroid injections, or just time – maybe a combination of all three – but eventually the pain subsided and I was able to get my life back.

I still have some pain but it is manageable. The anesthesiologist who did the steroid injections suggested some posture alignment work might be good for me, so I take a posture alignment/yoga class that has really helped not only my neck but my overall health as well.

In the past, when family members or friends experienced pain, I was always supportive and genuinely felt bad for them. I thought I was empathic. But until I had severe pain myself, I didn't really get what it was like for them.

> Because of this experience, I came to understand how someone in terrible pain would do virtually anything to make it stop.

My every waking moment was focused on the pain and wanting it to go away. I couldn't think about or concentrate on anything else. It makes sense to me that someone in such horrendous pain might first drink some alcohol to numb the pain. Then, if that didn't work, they might take some pain pills. When that was not enough, they might take more and more pills, hoping to see some relief. How easy it would be to overdose. The desperation caused by extreme pain is a slippery slope that so easily leads to disaster.

Luckily for me, my pain subsided to a level that I can live with. I don't know how those living with chronic, debilitating pain carry on. I guess they are also hoping that something, somehow, will make the pain go away.

* * *

4. Thirty Years A Slave to Pain

Workplace Accident: Rick

Thirty years ago, I fell forty feet from a roof. I was not expected to live. I had massive internal and orthopedic injuries, primarily on my right side. I spent about six weeks in intensive care just at the time they had started introducing trauma centers in hospitals. Without this, I probably would not have lived.

I was on a ventilator, draining tubes, and all kinds of gizmos. I went in and out of consciousness due in part to the heavy narcotics they had me on. My girlfriend (now my wife) was advised on a daily basis that I might not make it.

After a couple of weeks, I came back to consciousness and became aware of the gravity of my situation. I had to undergo multiple surgeries and gradually began to improve over the next six to eight weeks.

I am convinced it was my sheer will to live that kept me going. That and the support I had from my girlfriend and relatives and the many friends who sent cards that were plastered all over the walls of my room. They gave me inspiration to live.

When I was finally released from hospital, I was bedridden for about two months and could do very little. Then I got to go back home to Idaho. Being with my sister and her family and reconnecting with old friends meant everything to me.

For the next two years, I went through extensive physical therapy and occupational therapy. Because of my injuries and my physical limitations, it was impossible for me to return to work as a carpenter. I had an 86% disability rating with work man's comp! I retrained as a construction estimator since I knew the construction business so well. Unfortunately, when my schooling ended and at the same time my workman's compensation was terminated, the economy was bad and I couldn't find work. I suspect that my medical condition played a major role in the fact that I was turned down for jobs.

In the course of my therapy, I had a doctor who put me on a narcotic and did not do a good job of monitoring the medication. I became emotionally and physically addicted to Vicodin. It was the beginning of a long battle to fight the addiction.[11]

Because I could not find work as an estimator but had to have work to survive, I went back to working as a carpenter. At first, it was really hard – especially with the moving and lifting that had been no problem before the accident. I simply had to come to terms with that.

From that point forward, I worked pretty much full time and would feel wasted and in pain at the end of each day. I did massive doses of Advil and heat packs. Over the next few years, I gravitated toward finishing work in cabinetry which turned out to be easier and more enjoyable. I discovered I was good at it too.

I've had a number of surgeries over the years including two shoulder surgeries, knee surgery and fusion on my neck due to the fall and the work I was doing. Things in my body were wearing out faster than they normally would.

---

[11]To put Rick's experience in context, consider the following quote from the article by Katherine Schreiber entitled *Addiction in America: A big problem is getting bigger,* Psychology Today, Special Edition, Sussex Publishers, New York, January/February 2015: "Approximately 21.6 million Americans over the age of 12 are dependent on some kind of substance. That's 8.2 percent of the population. And nearly three quarters of involved individuals (15.3 million) are hooked on prescription drugs – the second most abused substance, after marijuana."

Then, about six years ago, I started developing sharp pains in my lower back – I mean, "bring-me-to-my-knees" pain where I literally could not stand up. This was when the real problems began.

I started back on painkillers and was keeping this a secret from my wife. I had to work, I justified to myself, and I kept on using for a couple of years. Finally, I went to a pain clinic and was able to wean myself off the medication for about six months.

Just getting out of bed was (and still is) a problem for me and I went back to using narcotics to cope, again without telling my wife. This issue put an enormous strain on our relationship over the years. She developed a level of distrust in me that was deeply disconcerting given that I am otherwise a very honest person.

I kept using for the next two years and wasn't focusing on finances. We got behind in our rent and were forced to move out of our home. For about six months we were homeless, staying in extended stay hotels and motels until we finally found a place to live. I understand how difficult it is to resist using drugs when you are in so much pain but I know from my own experience, they cause more problems than they're worth.

About a year ago, I went to see Dr. Frawley, a neurologist in Santa Barbara, and he immediately took me off Norco and put me on Suboxone. While I had not felt driven and desperate to get drugs at all cost, the body develops a dependence during continued use. The goal of the treatment was to block the high of narcotics but it also brought with it a lot of unpleasant side effects such as stomach problems, blocked libido and sweating profusely all of a sudden. I am tapering off Suboxone at the present, hoping I will not resume taking narcotics despite the ongoing constant pain. I have been to numerous physical therapists and even acupuncture but so far nothing works except the painkillers. It is a tough battle for me.

I try to be smarter about what I do at work but sometimes I have no choice. Then I pay for it later. Being tough is how I was raised and it's just the kind of guy I am.

> When I'm engaged in my work, sometimes I can forget about the pain. Then I drive home and can't get out of my car.

I've noticed that under life's stresses – for example my wife's brain tumor – my use of pain pills went up. But I've learned that reaching for the bottle is not as helpful as it may seem in the moment. There have been times where I felt hopeless and came close to suicide. In the end, I would never do that to my family.

I'm closing in on thirty years of this enslavement to pain and it is not an easy path. Just the same, I feel fortunate that I've made it this far despite all I've been through. They thought I would die but here I am, thirty years later, alive and hopeful. I am winning the battle after all.

*   *   *

5. The Way Out Is The Way In

Sports Accident: Wendy Allen, Ph.D, MFT

I have chronic pain because I was in a sports-related accident thirteen years ago. I was competing for points at a final event in a horse-jumping series. I had just completed a practice jump on my horse. Then, when my horse turned right, I turned left – right into the sand of the practice ring. This sort of fall happens all the time and the rider usually gets up, dusts the sand off her bottom, and gets back on the horse. I must have landed on my leg in some flukey way. There I was face down in the dirt and not able to move.

I remember yelling at the paramedics not to cut my formal riding boot off because these boots were among the most expensive wardrobe items I owned. The paramedics carried me on a stretcher face down. Only when we were in the hospital did they decide they had to turn me over. I begged them not to but they went ahead and did so. I heard someone screaming: "Please help me! Somebody help me!" The person screaming was *me*. Even with the powerful drug they gave me afterward, this marked the beginning of my life with chronic pain.

The irony was: I had enough points to win the series without going into the ring. I didn't even have to ride that day.

I had a compound fracture of my leg. They installed a titanium pole that was screwed into my femur that I named "Thor" because it held up my world ... kind of. Either the break or the operation – I'm not sure which – led to an RSD[12]

---

[12] Reflexive Sympathetic Dystrophy now known as Chronic Pain Pervasive Syndrome.

condition in my foot that was intense. When it flared up, I felt like my foot was *on fire*.

That accident changed my life. Always athletic and on the move, I became severely limited in what I could do with my body. I was confined to my hospital bed for a year and the solitude and inactivity drove my anxious self crazy.

> The doctors told me that I might never be able to walk normally again. At that point, I made the all-important decision that I was going to make my life better. I could not see myself stuck in a wheelchair or using a walker or crutches for the rest of my life. All these devices would only be temporary resources to help me get better. I was going to do whatever it took to walk normally and have less pain.

Thirteen years later, I am still on painkillers but I have gone from three a day to one-half. Weaning down on Vicodin is an insidious process but I managed because I told myself: "The way out is the way in" – that is to say, I got into this mess as an athlete and that's how I'm going to get out of it!

Being on even this low a level of painkiller still puts me under the new, rigid, so-called "bad-person" FDA regulations. I try not to mind.

Chronic pain is confusing. It means many things to many people. However, I have found that people who were in catastrophic accidents often tell a story remarkably close to mine.

1. An appetite and chronic pain can't co-exist. I lost twenty pounds. A woman I know lost forty.

2. The body naturally wants to shrink away from the pain. There is a mistaken yet compelling belief that if you get smaller, the body might hurt less.

3. Chronic pain sucks a lot of energy. Only now, thirteen years later, am I able to stand for two hours at a gathering or party. That is a huge victory. I can have a social life.

4. My chronic pain status could easily have become my lead in every conversation. I kept a lot to myself in silence.

5. Chronic pain can have a heavy impact on your spouse and family if you let it. I tried hard not to let it.

6. Chronic pain taught me lessons about patience, sustaining a vision, setting reasonable goals, and being my own cheerleader.

7. I learned I could be stoic and, in the words of my sister, was "as tough as nails." I like that description.

In the end, there is no happy silver lining to a chronic pain experience. The truth is: it is much better not to have it. But since we don't have a choice, let me tell you a little about my experience.

Recovery takes a long, long time. During that very stressful first year, my husband and I both had to learn to keep our ridiculous resentments in check and to ourselves. I was resentful because he could not read my mind and help me as I needed. He resented the burden he had to attend to before and after his work day.

I practiced what A.A. had taught me about handling resentments – to see what was under my resentment towards him. It was always my anger at the pain. I learned to get a grip on that and not go after him. Or at least keep it to myself until the mean thoughts passed.

I encouraged my husband to take piloting lessons, a dream he had had for a long time. It gave him something fun to do outside the home, something other than just work at the office and then work at home. In these ways both our resentments were addressed.

During that first year, I figured out a way I thought we could have sex. It involved a kitchen table. With my nightgown up around my waist, my husband could see for the first time the effects of the degrading, rapid deterioration of my left leg. My husband was so shaken and appalled, he could not perform. He was racked with guilt. I was humiliated.

I knew right away this would be a turning point for us. I could not let it end in failure and hurt feelings. In some inspired way, I said: "I'm still hot for you. Let's just get into the hospital bed together." We found a way! I am as proud of that moment as I am of almost anything.

My chronic pain is still with me. It makes me tired and lets me know when I've pushed too hard. Yet it is not at a level 10 anymore, more at a level 4. It is not now what defines me.

I cannot bend my injured leg in a regular sitting position for very long before it starts to hurt. At home I have two Lazyboys (and I am much too young for a Lazyboy.) The decorating theme of my home is comfort. A recent guest complained that she could get out of one of our overstuffed couches.

My husband and I have made a lifestyle out of celebrating my small physical victories.

I vividly remember the first time I could make my dinner without having to sit down and rest as I worked in the kitchen.

I remember the first time I could sleep on my left side. Changing positions in bed at night is a blissful experience. The year 2014 (thirteen years later) was the first time I could sit with my legs crossed, Indian style. I showed off that simple posture to anyone who would watch. Getting to have two ways to sit is really comfortable.

When we fly to see my family back East, I have to buy three seats so I can stretch out my left leg. That gets pricey! When we go to the movies, I bring a makeshift "ottoman" to use. Someone compliments me on it every single time saying:"Wish I had thought of that!"

I won't ever dance again. I can't run around with the dogs on the lawn.Yet, I can take them for a walk for 45 minutes now.

I owe my recovery success to Pilates, which has really been an advanced physical therapy for me. Pilates is hard and painful.This is where athleticism comes in. Hard and painful is absolutely worth it when I can see a result, any kind of improvement.

I see myself doing Pilates for the rest of my life. It is fascinating and varied and, I believe it will keep me interested for a long, long, time.At the same time it is keeping me out of the all-consuming chronic pain I lived in for many years.

I have a disability and always will, but I can do more and more stuff with my body and energy year after year.

My scar where they put Thor into me has faded a reasonable amount.Thor will be with me forever. It has made my left leg shorter than my right.

I have gained back half the weight I lost. I feel that my skinniness is my scar. I watch other skinny people now to see if they limp.

I am aware and proud of all my achievements through this time. Other people in my life, including my husband, are beginning to forget and that is how it should be. I won't forget.

I am a tough, stoic, athletic broad of 62, not too different from who I was before, yet, at the same time, utterly changed.

* * *

6. A Third of My Life

Migraine Headaches: Pete

My first memory of it was at age ten. In the backseat, lights coursing overhead as my father drove like a mad man through the winter night, on icy, treacherous roads to my uncle's. Late as usual. Around the same time, I was hit square in the face with a fully swung baseball bat. Not an assault, a mistake.

Whether it's stress or food related, I don't know, but fifty-eight years later, they're still with me: blinding migraines that usually last ten days to two weeks, and when I was much younger, as long as three weeks. Without interruption, forcing me to smash the right side of my head against a wall, just to relieve the pain from the left side, behind my eye.

Trauma work has changed nothing. Every test that could be taken has been taken. Every food that might trigger the headaches (sugar, chocolate, peppermint, alcohol, etc.) has been removed. Discussions with other migraine sufferers, comparing events, diets, medicines, acupuncture and therapies, continue. The headaches remain.

Otherwise, I *never* get sick.

Bright light can bring it on, and once the headache has bloomed, light is to be avoided. The prescription medications, like Cafergot and Imitrex, do not work. An acupuncturist, hoping to change the neural pathways, suggested no medication of any sort for two years. Break the cycle, he said. I lasted twenty months, the pain worse than ever. Now it's Extra Strength Tylenol, followed four or five hours later by 600mg of

Ibuprofen, followed four hours later by Vicodin. Then start the medicine cycle over again. All destructive to kidney and liver but essential for survival.

A stupor takes over me. The pain—always in the same place, behind and to the side of my left eye—churns like a bag of small rocks against my left occipital lobe and up to the optic nerve, then drills into the area left of my nose, an area called the lacrimal sac. It makes me ultra-sensitive, not only to light but to sound and touch and even smell, especially unnatural ones like perfumes and other chemicals.

With touch often unbearable, my wife is driven away, unless she gently massages my scalp. She's angry with me for "not taking care of myself." But what does that mean?

> Friends are helpless and who can blame them for turning away during these moments. No one wants to even think about pain.

So I get testy and insular. And, eventually, marginally depressed, though I've learned not to make any important decisions during these bouts of pain. The drill bit keeps turning in my eye, waking me out of a sound sleep or persisting through a daylong business meeting in a conference room. Rarely does anyone know but my wife, my family or my best friends. I just keep rubbing my head and downing pills. For an hour or two or three, I feel fine again. Not normal because I'm on edge, but pain-free. It returns.

I get cold, especially my fingers and toes. My scalp wants to lift off for outer space. My teeth ache. Sometimes if I've taken medication for a week or more, one of my inner ears hurt. And by the second week I can get restless leg syndrome, probably from the medication.

Lately, at the onset of the headache, I've tried Himalayan Crystal Salt in warm water with lemon juice. Remarkably, this drink almost immediately takes away the pain, though it can be hard on the stomach. Unfortunately, the pain tends to return in three or four hours, and may lose its impact after a couple days of use. But the concoction is certainly healthier on my body than the drugs.

I thought I'd grow out of the headaches. Other migraine sufferers have and there was a period of four to five years in which the headaches suddenly disappeared, though no conditions had changed. But they returned. One of my older clients, many years ago, had them *daily* his entire life. This could have been my fate, so I consider myself lucky. Two-thirds of my life is pain free. I've learned to relish those days.

Chronic pain is a condition that many humans experience, especially as we age. Though I still curse the pain, I find it remarkable how we learn to live with it (if we must).

It is a very personal space, not easily understood. For anyone who has not experienced extended pain, I suggest trying to find compassion for those who do, and that means foregoing blame or fear, and providing the person in pain with as much support and *benevolent space* as they need. Usually, that's all we can ask.

* * *

7. Just Breathe

Leukemia: Nancy Monnie

It is not enough for me just to be alive but I want to live.

I don't normally talk much about the pain I have experienced with Leukemia so I am not sure where to begin. As I look back on my life, I consider myself to have lived quite a privileged life overall. I have been extremely healthy and physically active my entire life. My body served me well for fifty-five years without any hitches. The only time I was in the hospital was to have my babies: totally natural childbirth without medication. I seldom took a pill of any kind and I seldom went to the doctor.

Amongst my friends I was the athletic one. I was running in the "fast lane of life," swimming competitively, playing on the high school softball team, participating in bike events, triathalons, runs, hikes, racquet ball, gymnastics, and other sports throughout the year. I loved to water ski at every opportunity. At the age of fourteen, I went to the Junior Olympics in Hawaii. I was determined to go to the competition and so did a lot of fundraising to get there.

I grew up extremely poor. We didn't have some of the things that people just take for granted such as a stereo, a television and, for a while, a car. As a side note, my friend actually gave me her bicycle after she won another bike at an amusement park. It was my prized possession for a long time.

My parents tried to support me in every way they could. The one lesson my dad taught me was how important it was to get an education. I knew that in order to rise above the poverty I was born into, I would need to do that very thing. First, I obtained my Bachelors degree at the University of Utah and then, some years later, I went on to college and received my Doctorate in Physical Therapy in 2003. Today I have my own physical therapy clinic with a pool site and a beautiful facility. It is my dream clinic which I love.

For fifty-five years my body served me well. Then I ran straight into a brick wall. I turned to the left but was met with a brick wall once again. I turned right and found the same outcome. There was no place to go.

When I was first diagnosed with Myelodysplastic Syndrome or MDS, I was feeling one hundred per cent, except for a mouth sore that had been present for four months. I have suffered with canker sores most my life, but finally decided to go to the doctor to see what was up. When the blood test came back, the doctors got concerned. A bone marrow biopsy showed that I did have a blood cancer called MDS. Ironically, the same week I was diagnosed, I had, in fact, been on a forty-seven mile bike ride. I was in great shape!

The doctors explained that treatment would require chemotherapy every month – consisting of two weeks where I would feel pretty lousy, one week where I would start to recuperate, and then the following week or so I'd be back in for another round. I just couldn't accept that as a life I so I refused treatment. When people would ask how I was doing, I would say, "For someone as sick as I am, I feel great."

One doctor told me that I had three to five years before it would very possibly turn into Acute Myeloid Leukemia or AML, a much more serious disease. Unfortunately for me, within a few months I found out I did have AML. I had no choice but to move forward in search of a bone marrow donor.

My oldest brother, sixty-three years old and in good health, though not a perfect match, was able to donate for me. He is definitely my hero.

There are gaps in my memory in dates and events when I was first hospitalized. I have been told that for several days, I was either awake and crying in pain, or I was "out" because of the strong's meds I was given. When my pain would elevate to a ten, I can only describe a feeling of all-consuming pain. It took all I had just to breathe. I did not communicate with anyone during those times and typically turned inward. I could hear the staff telling me to take slow deep breaths. I did my best to adhere to that command, but it wasn't easy. Sometimes squeezing someone's hand helped. The worst part was not knowing when and how intense the next episode might be. When it comes on, I just close my eyes and tell myself over and over to *just breathe.*

I do have some residual graft versus host disease, a condition more likely to happen when there is not a perfect match. I have also had multiple complications and setbacks. I have had five compression fractures in my thoracic spine with subsequent kyphoplasties where they shoot cement into the spine to help raise the vertebrae to maintain height. I have what is called "prednisone skin" meaning that I bruise or cut very easily. Just reaching into the refrigerator, I bumped the side of the door and sure enough was bleeding from that. I usually have bruises all over my elbows and the backs of my hands. I have been so weak at times that I can barely put one foot in front of the other the fatigue has been so extreme. Some of this can be a result of the medication.

I try to stay as active as I can and rode on my bicycle on a trail near our home in October. Without thinking, I put my bike shoes on and ended up not being able to get out of them quickly enough before I lost my balance and tipped over. Because of the prednisone, I have developed osteoporosis and so the fall caused a fracture at the neck of the femur. I had surgery the following day with four screws implanted. That was in October of 2014. I am now walking independently or with a cane. I use the cane when I'm at work in an effort to preserve energy for the hours that I am there.

Because the prednisone has caused cataracts in both my eyes, I am expecting to need cataract surgery. It is very difficult to see presently and it also affects my depth perception. This really makes a big difference in terms of managing my balance. As you can probably tell by now, I feel like I'm in this vicious cycle that never ends. In fact, later today I have an appointment to have the lesion on the side of my tongue biopsied. It seems so ironic to me that the mouth sore was what started this whole cycle in the spring of 2013.

There are times when I cope with this better than others. I can tell you that a lot of tears have been shed as I grieve and sorely miss the life that I once had. I am not a very patient person and as this goes on, it becomes more and more difficult to stay positive.

One has to hold on to hope and I do try to remain optimistic and to push myself as much as I can. I don't know how many people would attempt to return to work all day Monday, Wednesday, and Friday, within six weeks of fracturing the femur. The orthopedist at the last check just told me: "Do what you're going to do." He made it sound like I would not ever be pain-free even for normal walking. I hope to prove him wrong by rehabbing my leg.

The most frustrating part for me has been losing my independence. I am a very independent individual and not being able to drive myself when and where I want or need to go is probably one of the hardest parts about this whole ordeal. I am lucky enough to have a very loving and supportive family. My spouse takes care of preparing my meds each week. While I have found that he cannot really relate to what is going on with me and where I am coming from, in other aspects he is so loving and will do anything for me. My middle daughter, Alexis, moved home from New York City where she was following her dream of acting and is now my caregiver. She is a natural at it and has such a talent for this type of work. I am indebted to her and she has seen me through the thick and the thin. My oldest daughter Michelle has flown home every chance she can get to be by my side and my third daughter, Mikayla, who is serving a mission in Canada for our church, communicates with us weekly through emails. She always sends her love.

I have had so much support from my church group or what we sometimes call "my ward family." Meals have been brought in, visits have been made, posters and cards have been sent and these gestures mean so much to me. Prayers have been offered on my behalf and are still being offered. I am so thankful for all of these many blessings in my life. I have learned alot about gratitude over the past year in terms of how compassionate others can be when you are down and out. I have so much to be thankful for and so, when the dark times come, I try to recall the positive moments.

I do think that it is important to get out of bed each day and get dressed. I make sure I put on make up and do my hair. Even if I have moon face from Prednisone, I can at least look as if I am put together. I have a lot of people comment: "But you look so good," or "You look better this time than when I saw you just three weeks ago." Those types of comments always make my day.

It is nice to have someone to talk to, but I don't like being lectured on all the things I need to do. I guess what I am trying to say is that I want to be treated as an adult, not a helpless child. Sometimes all I want is a listening ear.

I do struggle with this new life. It is not enough for me just to be alive but I want to *live*. That is why I swam across the

Columbia River on Labor Day of 2013, just shy of twelve months post-transplant. That is why I jumped across a ditch to reach an elderly man who was about to collapse after crashing his car into a small tree. Unfortunately, I was not strong enough myself to help him, so both of us ended sitting in the grass waiting for someone to come to our rescue. That is why I got on my bicycle. That is why I returned to work post femur fracture. I can understand now why we read about people climbing Mt. Everest after a bout with cancer or some other dreaded disease. They want to feel alive once again. I am not planning anything that drastic, but kudos to those who are brave enough to do so.

For me the journey continues. I still crave the life I once had. I still hope I can get it back. I am learning patience the hard way. I wish I could tell you that all of this is past tense, but I am still very much in the middle of this ongoing horrific treatment. Today, in fact, I went to the eye doctor in the a.m. and to the oral surgeon in the p.m. with a biopsy of a lesion on the side of my tongue. I now have stitches on my tongue. I plan to go to work tomorrow, because staying busy is best for my body and my psyche. I carry on because that is who I am. I always remind myself to *just breathe.*

*   *   *

8. Elevator Ride with Pain

I. Open Heart Surgeries: Otis

Heart Pain

Pain from my perspective has always been relative – that is, compared to other pain experienced over my lifetime. A companion of pain is "hurt," sometimes indistinguishable, often difficult to define or categorize, but nevertheless quite real.

I have had two open heart surgeries, one in 2001 and the other in 2006. Prior to 2001, I was in a hospital only once for a few days when I was seventeen for the removal of a hemangioma from the bottom of my foot. When that tumored blood vessel acted up, I could barely walk. The pain level was a 10 and brought tears to my eyes. There were no tears either before or after both valve replacements.

The journey to my first heart surgery began in January 1989 with a diagnosis of a "leaky" aortic valve that would eventually have to be replaced. The trick was to wait long enough to catch the erosion of the value's efficacy before it tore away from the heart allowing blood to cascade out of the heart and kill me before I hit the floor. Annual physicals became de rigor.

In August 2001, my primary care physician advised me that I had "a *really* leaky valve." It was time. About five weeks later, I was on an operating table getting a mechanical aortic valve as opposed to a "tissue" valve (commonly referred to as a "pig" valve) on the theory that, ironically, I only wanted to do this once.

I woke up in a recovery room wondering what ran over me. Then I was scooted off to ICU for a few days for close monitoring of my body's acceptance of the valve, my pain levels and my blood clotting time. Patients are asked to judge their pain levels on a scale of 1 to 10 so that their pain meds can be adjusted. I have no recollection of ever saying "10" but I sure as hell know there were no "1's" or "2's" prior to discharge. People in less pain allegedly heal more rapidly and people differ in their pain tolerance threshold.

Participation in a cardio-vascular rehabilitation program after heart surgery was an essential key to regaining strength physically and mentally by watching my own as well as others' daily improvement. The most pain came when a nurse did a "finger stick" to draw a small amount of blood in order to check my blood clotting time. Although a finger stick became a routine over these last thirteen years, I do not look forward to having the tip of my finger poked with a tiny blade. It *hurts*, albeit temporarily.

In October 2006, my annual echo cardiogram discovered an aneurism in my ascending aorta. Damn! Here we go again. The mechanical valve was fine. Supposedly they are good for twenty years or more but the data is somewhat fuzzy because people may die of something else before the mechanical valve would ever wear out. I looked at the prospect of having a second open heart surgery as something of a good news/bad news story: I knew what to expect. Or so I thought.

This time was different. Three inches of my ascending aorta had to be removed along with the first mechanical valve. A unitary piece consisting of a new mechanical valve and three inches of what I believe is Teflon tubing or Teflon-like material was sutured back on to the heart and aorta. This was a more complex operation than heart surgery #1, with more pain, more hurt, and a little longer recovery period. More pain was due to an incision on the inside top of my left leg at about the entry point for an angiogram. It hurt like hell any time I moved.

On the second or third day post ICU, sometime around 5a.m., I decoupled myself from the medical equipment, wandered out into the hall and began shouting for everyone to leave because the hospital was closing and the nurses had lost their jobs. (Was this a flashback to a time when I actually had to go close one of our chemical plants?) Drugs can make you do strange things. A massive bruise appeared on the left side of my chest, rib cage and stomach area immediately after this episode. I was almost as zonked out the remainder of that day as Janis Joplin must have been when she checked out of this world. And I was at least a "9" for the next couple of days. Neither the bruising nor the severe pain had occurred in 2001.

Pain meds have a proclivity to cause constipation, which for me, caused pain more real than imagined until the magical event occurred some days later clearing both bowel and brain of pain.

An integral part of my recovery process, as well as diminution of pain, was my choice to continue my consulting practice.

> One of the paths to full recovery, in my opinion, is getting back into whatever you like doing rather than sitting around feeling sorry for yourself or dwelling on pain that may last longer than anyone foretold or expected.

If you are in business for yourself, you will be back at it sooner than you think. Retired? A volunteer? Don't want to go back to your job until you absolutely have to? If you read the classics or the biographies of successful people, you will find that being useful, productive and intellectually engaged is excellent therapy. It will help you heal.

As mentioned earlier, pain and hurt are relative phenomena. Heart surgery #2 was more painful than heart surgery #1 but neither was as severe as the periodic pain pulses of the tumored blood vessel that occurred over several months when I was seventeen years of age.

II. Otis: Prostate Cancer

Cancer Pain

There was both cancer and cardiovascular disease in my family history. Prior to 1989, I used to joke that I had a 50/50 chance of getting one or the other. I now knew my long term fate – heart disease. That all changed in 2009 when my PSA graph started to resemble a hockey stick. A biopsy confirmed prostate cancer. Now I had a real pain in the ass, and in the busiest year of my practice ever. Now what was I to do?

With a leaky heart valve, the options are pretty simple: do the surgery with low odds of dying on the table (age is a big factor) or forego the surgery and know that you will die. It's a simple choice. With prostate cancer, however, there are various alternatives. I read up on them all, hoping that one would jump off the page and say "I'm the one for you, baby!" Unfortunately, all were fraught with the potential for nasty collateral damage and there was a real probability that whatever procedure was elected, not all the cancer would be eliminated. Surgeons want to operate, radiologists want to radiate, and oncologists want to do chemotherapy. I concluded there were no all-good alternatives. All prostate cancer options have pros and cons. Not all successful outcomes are equal.

Collateral damage can be heinous. Place your bets and take your chances. But first, be sure to check your doctor's litigation track record.

Based on my research, I succumbed to the marketing hype of robotic surgery: shorter hospital stay = one day, less loss of blood, and overall quicker recovery time. I decided to have a urologist use the Da Vinci robot believing I could get back to work sooner and the cancer would be gone – at least the way he explained it. The best laid plans… The pain and hurt I was about to incur and endure for the next several months as direct result of this botched surgery made all prior (and subsequent) pain levels pale in comparison and duration.

My wife and I met with the surgeon. He seemed annoyed by some of my questions. There were a number of questions I never got to ask because he cut our meeting short. He was busy – so was I. I mistook his cockiness for competence. My wife took an immediate dislike to him. I should have paid attention to her sound judgment. When I asked how many prostatectomies using the Da Vinci robot he had performed, he said 170. After my surgery, I am of the opinion the actual number performed would be closer to the number 7 than the number 170. Unfortunately, there is often no way of verifying what a doctor tells you. A clinic or a hospital is not going to give you any information on prior cases or outcomes short of litigation. Then it's too late.

My research did not go far enough. I did not go to the courthouse to see if he had been sued for malpractice in our county. Big mistake. Had I become aware of the malpractice lawsuits filed against him, I would never have let that guy touch me.

Monday night before the surgery, I stayed in a hotel within walking distance of the hospital. I couldn't eat even a light dinner. I had trouble sleeping. Walking to the hospital in the dark at 5:00 that Tuesday morning, I understood why some people cancel their scheduled surgeries: they may well be too frightened. A fear of the unknown is real. I had bad vibes about this one.

The day after surgery, I was released to go home. I felt really awful. It was painful walking, sitting, standing, and lying down. A catheter hookup was a new and clumsy experience. Something inside did not feel quite right, but I could not pinpoint where or what. I did not anticipate such a high level of pain (8-9) and bodily hurt after this surgery. Nor did I feel any better on the third and fourth day home. I actually thought I was getting worse. On Saturday I called the clinic. The urologist on call said there was nothing he could do because the clinic was closed. "Go to urgent care or the emergency room" was his advice. Welcome to the modern medical practice style.

Urgent care couldn't figure out what was wrong with me. I was sent home only to wait to go to the ER on Monday morning. There I passed a substantial amount of blood and was readmitted to the hospital. My pain was at a 10. I had developed a grayish pallor, looking like death warmed over, and for the first time in my life, I thought I was going to die. Was an Obama death panel in my immediate future?

I was in a world of hurt. It did not help matters that my urologist looked and acted panic-stricken as he told my wife and I that they were going to find out what was wrong with me. The surgery was, after all, successful? Right? So much for a shorter hospital stay and quicker recovery.

No one at the hospital could figure out what was wrong with me. Despite a myriad of x-rays, CT scans, MRI's, blood tests, urine analyses and who knows what else over the next six days, either a sigmoidoscopy and or a colonoscopy had to be performed amid the sewage cesspool my colon, rectum and bowel had become. Finally, ten days after the surgery, the gastroenterologist located the problem: a puncture wound in my anterior rectum that could only have come from the botched surgery at the hands of my urologist. A general surgeon then performed a colostomy, a word never before in my lexicon. These two surgeons saved my life that day. It was Friday the 13th.

The "Operative Report" for the colostomy reads in part: "Upon opening the abdomen, a large amount of blood was evacuated. Approximately 600-700 ml. of blood and clots were removed from the abdomen… The pelvis was inspected. There was noted to be stool as well as fecal material with old blood in the pelvis…" I now know why I was at a "10".

Upon gaining some modest level of consciousness in Recovery, I could not fathom what had taken place. I did not comprehend colostomy or even know how to pronounce it. Shortly after migrating to ICU, I got to observe the colostomy incision when the wound dressing was being changed. It was with shock and horror that I looked at the length (navel to pelvis), depth and width of the open wound. It was as if I went in for an appendectomy and they amputated my arm. And what the hell was that bag attached to a new hole in the left side of my abdomen? I was an "8-10" for several days. My "hurt" was a "10."

After the colostomy and while I was in ICU, the meds caused me to hallucinate but it was different from the episode after my second heart surgery. This time around, I saw extremely bright lights, colorful, flashing, rotating, spinning lights. I heard a bus making a high pitched idling noise just outside my room. After I could not get a nurse to attend to my ostomy seal, I became convinced that those travel nurses were going to kill me. Did they drop some acid on me? Was I losing my mind? I had to get out of there. The next morning when my cardiologist made his rounds to check on my blood clotting time, I begged him to get me out of there and up to a room on a floor. He did. I began to feel better almost immediately. I was grateful.

My next office visit with him was after my Echo in October 2010 when he complimented me on my recovery, and what was a first for him – a patient who made it through ICU four times! Sweet.

It was after lunch on Thanksgiving Day that I was finally discharged, 22 days after the prostatectomy and 12 days after the colostomy. I was home at last. I could rest. I could get some sleep. A hospital may not be the ideal place to be when you are sick or recovering from surgery. In a word? Noise! Beginning early in the morning with a blood draw, the discordant noise rages on nearly 24/7 from shift changes, to meals being served, to a gaggle of interns and residents observing, assisting, asking questions, to M.D.'s making their rounds, to the do-gooders visiting. It seems as if nobody is on the same schedule. Why do families and friends think this is a social occasion and party time? Why are kids under twelve allowed on the floor? Don't other patients get exhausted from entertaining family and friends?

Sleep deprivation takes its toll. Sleeping for me masked the pain and the hurt if only for short flashes of time.

> Had the police presented me with a list of unsolved crimes dating back to Christ, I would have confessed to them all in return for some quiet place to sleep.

During this hospital stay, my wife was given a couple of training sessions on how to change the dressing and treat the wound. We still joke about the fact she virtually became an Ostomy nurse on sixty minutes of training. Nonetheless, it was sufficient in combination with assistance from Visiting Nurses and the nurse for the surgeon who performed the colostomy. I thank God for being blessed with a loving, caring wife who stepped up to the challenge of caregiver – not only for this ordeal but also for the two heart surgeries, the prostatectomy, the colostomy and the fifth surgery five months later to reverse the colostomy, I would never have made it without her.

A colostomy is something I would not wish upon anyone. God bless those who have adjusted well enough to lead normal lives while wearing an ostomy bag. The video I was shown depicts people of various ages, kids to mature adults, male and female, running, swimming, playing tennis, working and otherwise leading normal day-to-day lives. For five months I wore an ostomy bag. At the beginning it was close to a living hell. It was better after I learned to adapt and accept the facts at hand. I became less self-conscious in a social setting but always remained somewhat uncomfortable for fear of a bag malfunction.

Since my rectum was "perforated" by the urologist, it needed to be kept clear of stool while the puncture wound healed. During a colostomy, part of the colon is connected to an opening (stoma) in the abdomen. This is where stool now leaves the body. Stool passes through the stoma into a special bag. Ostomy bags have seals that fit around the stoma so that fecal matter can be excreted into the bag that attaches to the seal affixed to the skin via an adhesive. Sometimes I got a complete seal to the skin, other times not. Sometimes a perfect seal would separate from the skin. In these cases, it was most disconcerting because I had no control over when my body was going to evacuate excrement. I had to change a lot of seals and bags.

The video portrayed changing the ostomy bag and the seal as a relatively simple process. If I was careful, the bag change became fairly easy. The seal not so. My skin has always been sensitive. Removing the seal was painful, at times reminding me of the hemangioma pain (a "10"). You don't take painkillers for transient pain of that kind. Often the pain lingered because my skin became so irritated. Lotions helped but did not cure. My skin never did become like Buffalo hide and thereby impervious to the pain. Not everyone is so adversely affected.

The puncture wound in the rectum finally healed in April 2010 and the colostomy was reversed. I marveled at how, during those five months, the colostomy surgical wound gradually closed from the navel to the pelvis, side to side, from the bottom of the incision up, leaving angry-looking scar tissue the length of the incision. I may have had some pain post reversal but I have no recall of anything significant during this final wound closing

Heart surgery #2 was a good news/bad news event: for the most part, I knew what to expect. For the prostatectomy, I thought I knew what to expect. I was anticipating some temporary issues but was completely unprepared for the resulting damage. If I had to do it over, I would go to a surgeon in a large hospital who performs robotic surgery routinely and has done lots of them. The colostomy surgery was absolutely necessary and, even knowing what I experienced over those five months, I would do it again provided there was no other remedy.

As a result of the colostomy, the lining in my abdomen was weakened. This later morphed into a hernia that no one wanted to operate on because of their concern that the lining and the mesh would not hold together. Incidentally, nation-wide litigation concerning mesh screen failures may also be a factor. Quite frankly, I'm not looking to have any more surgeries. If the hernia becomes strangulated, I'll go ahead with surgery if it can be done. Otherwise, it will be time to finish getting my affairs in order. At present, another surgery is not something I give thought to.

Nevertheless, adding insult to injury, I still have prostate cancer, now treated every six months by chemotherapy.

It seems a tad strange that a drug can beat a PSA level down to undetectable levels, only to have it rise back up after six months to a level requiring another dose to knock it down again. We can't kill the steely beast! I wonder if the drug manufacturers could tweak the formula to become a permanent fix rather than a repetitive long term treatment. A magic bullet so to speak. You think? I wish.

Ironically, I do not think of myself as having cancer, nor do I dwell on it. The cancer, wherever it is in my body, causes no pain. A cancer patient I knew summed it up: "If it wasn't this, it'd be something else." We both agreed with W.C. Fields that on the whole we would rather be in Philadelphia.

Afterthought

When I read through this story, I had the thought that someone might read this and say: "This guy is a complete mess!" That is not at all true. Of the many challenges in life, some are more complex than others. Here in early 2015, I am still off the elevator of pain and can live with what I have been dealt. The aches and pains are age-related. The hurt has vanished. I am content.

*　*　*

9. The Body Remembers

Ectopic Pregnancy: Louise Currey

It was all reduced to this intense pain with no beginning, no end, no reason, and no resolution. It filled every crack of my being leaving no space for anything else. Life itself did not matter.

When I was seventeen, married two years and the mother of a one-and-a half-year-old little boy, our little family moved to West Los Angeles from the east coast. No sooner did we arrive than I became pregnant, an unplanned but not unhappy event. My husband, age 28 when I married him at age 15, had asked that I postpone my education until we had children because he did not want to be an "old father" as his own had been. I agreed as he said he would support my education once our family was under way.

Things were uneventful for the first five or six weeks as we settled in. We had only one car so walking was how I got around while he was at work. One morning I placed my son Bobby in the stroller to go to the market for groceries, a walk we both thoroughly enjoyed. In the market, I felt a wave of nausea and said to myself "uh oh, morning sickness." The feeling quickly passed. Then I felt a new feeling – things went black and I swayed with dizziness, struggling to remain conscious and staggering to stay upright. "Help!" I shouted to a clerk. "I'm pregnant and I need to sit down. I'm about to pass out. Where can I sit? Please watch my son!" The clerk pushed a carton of canned goods my way and I collapsed with my head between my knees.

I don't know how long I sat there but the dizziness passed eventually, only to be replaced by a weariness so intense I could barely rise to my feet. The walk home, only four or five blocks, seemed eternal. I remember thinking "One foot in front of the other. Concentrate. You can't go to sleep on the sidewalk. What about Bobby?" Thank goodness I had him harnessed securely in his stroller and the walk was making him drowsy because he was such a wiggly worm.

I decided to stop for help at my friend Eileen's apartment one building over from mine. I rang her bell pleading: "Eileen, can you help me? I almost fainted in the market. I don't know what's wrong with me. I'm so exhausted." She took the groceries and my son plus stroller upstairs to my apartment while I very slowly climbed the stairs using my arms as much as my legs. My feet felt like stone and I had to will myself to the top. I collapsed in my bed and fell asleep immediately.

For the next five or six weeks, I was moving in slow motion and unable to think clearly. Everything was an effort. I would stagger lifting Bobby to the changing table or high chair. I felt sharp spreading pain whenever he bumped my stomach, but it did not register with me that this was so much different from my first pregnancy. In retrospect, this pain was an important symptom that the doctor missed also. It was much later that I learned that the pain was indicative of "guarding," a medical term for inflammation of the peritoneal cavity – often from internal bleeding. I was too dulled in my thinking to report this finding to the doctor and he did not test my abdomen for guarding. The lethargy continued.

Then I could not eat. I could not keep down any solid food beyond a cup of thin oatmeal gruel per day and sugared tea to keep myself hydrated. Making it to the bathroom grasping on to furniture took all my energy and left me gasping. I could only shower once a week with help to stand up.

The pain was like peristalsis magnified one hundred times. It was a smooth muscle pain more intense than labor pain and similar to passing a kidney stone but, in my case, it never stopped for three whole months! As it swept over me, it heightened my hearing so that every sound was intensified. The apartment building seemed to creak and groan. Footsteps on the stairs and even on the pavement below pounded in my head. The wood frame of the apartment came alive, breathing and wheezing. The wind seemed to cry. Could I really hear my neighbors talking in the next building? Could my husband's footsteps on the carpet sound like crunching leaves?

The center of my universe was the pain in my belly. It left no room for any other experience. Hate, love, reason, joy, hunger, worry – none of this mattered. Day, night, midday – it did not matter. My husband, my son, even I myself – did not matter. It was all reduced to this intense pain with no beginning, no end, no reason, and no resolution. It filled every crack of my being leaving no space for anything else. Life itself did not matter.

Then the doctor began making home visits to administer morphine injections. For four hours a day, I had some relief of pain and I could sleep.

> My whole being became focused on the arrival of the needle with the precious morphine that would release me from the pain that sliced my body into fillets.

One day, I recall, a thought sailed by as I became aware of how focused I was on that needle. "Now I know what it is like to be an addict."

Incredibly, I spent three months on total bed rest unable to move, think, help myself or help my son. It was not until a wave of nausea led me to ask the doctor for a basin into which I vomited green bile that he woke up to the gravity of my situation. Green bile is not produced from the stomach but from intestinal contents further along and it cannot be produced voluntarily. The doctor said: "I want to hospitalize you. You have lost forty pounds and this green bile suggests intestinal blockage. I'll talk with your husband about getting you admitted into L.A. County General. At six months pregnant, an abdominal surgery requires an obstetric specialist." I felt profound relief that finally I was being taken seriously. I had been too weak and frail to fight to get the proper care for myself. Somehow my body provided the proof the doctor needed to recognize a life-threatening condition.

L.A. County General is a teaching hospital. I had six complete physical examinations including one with a doctor who had never done a pelvic exam before – and admitted it to me. Full of morphine, I felt generous and reassured him that I had had many pelvics before and they didn't bother me. He survived.

They left my chart at my bedside and I read the findings each student had noted including their putative diagnoses. Of the six, only one was correct.

Off to surgery. I was given a local anesthesia, a caudal block, because of my unborn baby. With the first incision – diagonal at my right abdomen – I felt the sensation of my skin parting but no pain. The surgeon used retractors to look into the abdomen. He looked up and said to the anesthesiologist: "Put her under." A hiss of gas through a face mask and I awakened in Recovery, my stomach strangely flat and bandaged. "What! No baby? What else is gone? Will I ever be able to have other children? Then I passed out again.

I woke up in a darkened room. Silhouetted in the doorway, my husband softly cried. This touched my heart. Until then, I had not been sure he loved me since expressing affection was hard for him. "I'm okay; we'll make it. I love you," I reassured him. Shock and anger came through his voice as he responded: "I almost lost you. I don't know how I would handle that! The doctor told me you were trying to get an abortion. He didn't know how sick you were. Can you imagine?"

We must keep in mind that this was the early fifties when abortions in the first trimester were illegal in California and doctors took god-like paternalistic stances especially with women, assuming they knew what we were thinking and what was best for us. Today, with some exceptions, doctors are more willing to be up-front and negotiable. Moreover, I am not the person I was at age seventeen. I would not be willing to contract with physicians who would be secretive and controlling in this way.

At that time, no one on the maternity ward would tell me what had happened. "The doctor will tell you soon" was the only answer I received. It was more than a day later when the chief surgeon came to my bedside. He was middle-aged, kind, and direct – just as a doctor should be. "You still have your appendix," he began. "Remember that when people ask you about your appendix scar. You were too sick for us to do an appendectomy. We delivered a baby boy weighing slightly over one pound. He is not expected to live. I am so very sorry." He paused and took my hand. "We had to deliver him because he was in your abdominal cavity and not in your womb. His arms and legs were tangled in your intestines. No wonder you were in such pain!" He paused again. "The placenta had attached itself to part of the right broad ligament that supports the uterus after the right fallopian tube ruptured." He shook his head. "It is a one in a million occurrence. I've only seen two live births like this in my forty-year obstetrical surgery career.

You will have adhesions but your uterus is intact and we were able to save your left ovary and tube. You will be able to have more pregnancies in the future if you wish."

Three days later, on a Sunday, I was visited by grief over the death of this little boy I never saw, never held, never kissed, and was unable to save. My milk came in and my breasts were hot and painful in the binder I had to wear. At the same time, I was experiencing morphine withdrawal. I sat in a window seat in that hospital high up in the clouds listening as organ music drifted up from the hospital chapel below and cried for it all.

A cluster of interns came in on rounds to view this unusual case. One young man asked me: "How did you deal with all that severe pain?" I didn't know how to answer. My tongue could not pull anything from my brain. Then this answer came out: "What else could I do? I could not escape it. The pain was my total existence."

When it was time for my sutures to come out and the doctor approached me with the sterile suture removal scissors, my belly went into involuntary tremors. "I'm so sorry, I can't make my stomach stop," I explained. My hands on my belly were no help. My body remembered the pain it had been through. I think it still does. The body does not forget.

* * *

10. Not an Easy Life

Brain Tumor: Justin

There were few students with conditions like mine because most patients with brain tumors died.

At four years of age, I was diagnosed with a tumor on the right side of my brain. It swelled to the point that it was cutting off the fluid from my spine. I had been complaining of headaches but no doctors listened to my mom. The tumor grew larger until the pressure was overwhelming. It took about four months for them to take us seriously. They finally identified the tumor and did surgery to remove it. They put in a shunt or pump that ran from my head into my neck. To make room for the shunt, they had to remove a sizable portion of my brain.

As a result, I had learning disabilities including a speech impediment and dyslexia. Also, I had to wear a helmet because if anyone hit the place on my head where the shunt was located, I would have died. As you can imagine, with all these cognitive difficulties as well as the all-too-conspicuous helmet I had to wear, I was constantly picked on at school. Children of that age, and even older, could not understand why I was so different.

I was placed in a special education class with a number of Down's Syndrome kids. Even though I didn't have this condition, I was treated the same as those who did. What was difficult was that I was aware of being an outcast whereas these children were not. Somewhere around this time, I started hiding the helmet because it made me feel like an oddball.

I also had epilepsy and was forced to take medication that speeded up my thoughts and made it hard for me to keep up. It made me feel like I was not myself. In third grade, I was held back while my twin sister got to go on to the next grade. She was always an A student and I felt compared all too unfavorably to her.

In fifth grade I discovered cannabis. It slowed down my brain so I could think more clearly. It really helped me. I got caught a few times for smoking weed but I kept using. I was skipped from Grade 5 to Grade 7 and was placed again in a special education class. There were few students with conditions like mine because most patients with brain tumors died. I had a really bad stuttering problem that got worse when I was nervous. Having teachers talk down to me didn't help. I felt that the school was trying to get rid of me.

In Grade 7, the shunt failed and I was rushed to Cottage Hospital. The surgeon tried to remove it and was unsuccessful. He just gave up on me and told my mother I was going to die. My mother drove frantically down to U.C.L.A. They threatened to arrest her for driving me and not using an ambulance but they gave up this idea when she arrived.

I died in the car on the way to the hospital. I saw a bright light and I was going through a tunnel toward the light. I woke up in an elevator at the hospital screaming to get out. A week later, I woke up with the shunt removed and more brain damage. I had that shunt from age four to age thirteen. My memory was affected and I felt like I had lost years of my life. But I survived. Of the three surgeries of this type the doctor had conducted, I was the only one to survive.

I failed Grade 8 so they skipped me to Grade 9 at Santa Barbara High School. In Grade 10, they moved me into a La Cuesta class primarily for troubled kids rather than those with Down's Syndrome. I pretty much learned on my own and felt that, for me, school was a waste of time.

My mother wanted me to get a job at age fifteen and couldn't understand why I was unable to find work. I couldn't live up to her standards. She sent me to my aunt's in Belize and I spent a year there. Things had changed on my return. She had left the stepfather I had been with since age three. [I never met my biological father.] My mother had started drinking again after eleven years of sobriety and my sisters were smoking in the house. It was a new world for me.

At seventeen, I was kicked out of continuation school with enough credits for a Grade 9 education. I never graduated as my sister did.

I met a girl ten years older than me and had a baby with her when I was nineteen. My mother disapproved but she was in the process of moving to New Mexico. I stayed with that woman for three years.

In February of 1991, I learned that my mother had hung herself. She had a history of suicide attempts – once she threw herself in a river and once she stabbed herself with a butcher knife. When she was suicidal, my sister and I were placed in a foster home. My mother's father and three sisters had all taken their own lives.

I carved my mother's name in my arm multiple times to release my pain. I was drinking and experimenting with every drug I could find. I wanted to be where my mother was. My mother had been a strict disciplinarian and used to hit me with a wooden spoon but she taught me right and wrong. She used to tell me she loved me many times a day. Without her, I was a lost soul.

> The day I got the news of my mother's suicide, my girlfriend broke up with me and took our baby with her. I had always dreamed of being in a family. She took away that dream.

In July of 1991, I was in a car accident. I was in a coma for about 2 weeks and had 185 stitches in my head. I hit the windshield and my right leg was crushed. They had to cut me out with the jaws of life. When I woke up the first time, I thought I was twelve years old. The second time I thought I was fifteen. My leg was in a cast and I was screaming. It turned out that my foot and ankle were crushed and my lower leg was broken in seven places. It healed wrong because they had set it the way it was and casted it. The surgery had to be redone.

In 1992, I broke my left leg from putting weight on it to avoid putting pressure on my other leg. I had to use crutches.

In 1994, I was walking in a crosswalk with a cane and was hit in a crosswalk by a city truck. Witnesses said I flew up twelve feet in the air and then came down on the pavement. This accident started a problem in my back and neck. When I went to court, the city said I was trying to kill myself and gave me minimal compensation for the accident.

I met another woman and moved with her to Paso Robles where we had my second daughter in 1998. I stayed home and raised her while her mother worked. Then we had my third daughter in 2000 and I raised her too. I quit drinking and went on prescription painkillers in high doses. In 2005, the relationship ended and I was separated from my daughters. I had a kind of nervous breakdown and cut my hand almost completely off. It was literally dangling from my arm. It took twelve hours of surgery to repair.

I was homeless for seven years, living in my van. I had night terrors and had to take a medication to stop from dreaming. I smoked marijuana morning, noon and night. In the van, unable to get a housing voucher, cold and wet, in severe pain and unable to get pain medication, I felt hopeless and wanted to die. Instead, I walked to the church up the street and my prayers were answered. The lady there gave me an apartment to live in – a home at long last.

Although I have a lot of pain, I am doing better now. Without help from doctors, I made a huge effort to cut down my pain medications. I managed to go from 600 mg of morphine down to 45 mg. I cut out Fentanyl, Methodone, Norco and Valium on my own. Despite my efforts to drastically reduce my medications, my doctor refused to honor his promise to refill my prescriptions. With three bulging discs in my neck and the pain in my leg, I was desperate. Dr. Bearman stepped in and saved my life. He has been like a father to me. It infuriates me that he has been judged for trying to help people like myself.

> Even though I have lowered my dosage, I am labeled everywhere I go as a drug seeker.

I am still being judged the same way I was ten years ago although I am on a fraction of the drugs. The little amounts I'm on now give me the same relief as the huge amounts I was on in the past. It's not for the purpose of altering mood; it's just to cope with life. To walk, to enjoy life, to have fun at all involves pain for me. When I go for help, I receive judgment in place of compassion.

I am with a new woman now in a loving relationship and I help her with her two children. When I met her, I wanted to cut out all my medication but I still need some to manage my life. I am happy now although I still have a lot of pain in my body. Love is what makes it possible to live my life.

*   *   *

11. Pain by Design

Shattered Ankle: David Eagle

I am a fifty-five year old single father of one beautiful twelve year old boy. Ten years ago in Oregon, I hopped off a wall about six feet above the ground. I had no idea that this one action would place me in an existential crisis without end. When I landed from the hop off the wall, I caught my left heel on the edge of a concrete slab below. My weight combined with my unfortunate landing changed everything from my perspective.

"Changed everything from my perspective" is not a characterization I could, or would, have articulated at the time of my accident. Yet I was changed the moment I landed.

When my left heel (calcaneus) hit the concrete slab, it shattered into 40+ pieces. The sideways momentum of my "hop" continued to rip my shattered heel completely out of the beautiful structure of bone which had cradled my ankle flawlessly from birth. Everything that structurally had been my left ankle was gone in that instant.

Time is perception. As I sat on the concrete, my cross-country running shoes were still on my feet. The athletic shoe I was wearing had very good support, so with the heavy wool hiking socks I was wearing, everything looked "normal" and in that moment I believed I had dodged another bullet. I was wrong.

When I tried to stand, the hope of escaping my fate vanished.

Within minutes my foot had swollen out of and around my left shoe. I remember that the friend I was with helped me to the car.

> Pain was still in the queue of trauma that was beginning to change my perception of everything without my permission.

We were staying at a hotel in Ashland, Oregon, and I remember my friend bringing a luggage cart to the truck and pushing me into the hotel elevator.

This is the depth of denial which trauma propagates. I had my friend drive me to our hotel, instead of the emergency room. In retrospect, I believe I realized the severity of my situation, but I was not ready to have it medically verified. After about an hour of feeling the pressure on my now ballooning left foot, pain began to whisper in my soul. I remember feeling as though my foot was taking on a life that was mine, and I would surely be lost.

Pain forced me to the Ashland Emergency Room. The ER technicians left my engorged foot in the sock and shoe to get some cursory X-Rays. The images were reflected in the surgeon's face. I asked the obvious: "So how bad is it?" The surgeon proceeded to describe the extent of the damage. The information was thready as I was now six hours post accident with no medical intervention. The surgeon kept stressing the need to get me into surgery. I finally asked, "What does all of this mean?" "Amputation" was the answer. Now I was present. I said, "No way are you cutting my foot off!"

The surgeon began to explain that I would never walk again, and in his opinion, I would be back within a year begging him to cut my foot off. I could not bring myself to intentionally amputate my left foot. I was rather attached to it. My rationale was that I could always amputate later. So against my surgeon's advice, I instructed him to put everything back as best he could to approximate an anatomically correct ankle. Ten hours later, I was in post-op and feeling no pain. For the next few days in the hospital, I had lots of morphine and support.

In an effort to streamline the spirit of this story, I will summarize the evolution of my ankle and my pain at that time. After the first surgery, I rejected the titanium plate on my heel, the numerous 2" screws, and even the "Bone-in-a-Bottle" used to fill in the lost bone. I went through a second surgery where everything was removed, and they left the wound open while they flowed a powerful antibiotic drip 24/7 over the exposed partial surgery. I remember at least five to ten days in this operative stasis before they sewed my foot back together, minus the hardware.

From accident to end of healing after the surgeries, took about three years. So the true nature of my initial decision NOT TO AMPUTATE was masked by the secondary trauma of surviving multiple surgeries. The truth is that I still had not "held" the full scope of my injury. I was on large amounts of morphine, so I had inadvertently created a three-year buffer between my perception and my actual physical state. Time is perception.

Five years post accident, I was still in a fog of drugs and pain. I was halfway through a doctoral program in Clinical Psychology when the accident occurred. I had to drop out of the program and lose my coursework. I still had not fully grasped the scope and breadth of my injury, although the permanence of my situation seemed inevitable. My son was two years old when I was injured. He spent the better part of his early childhood experiencing his father in agony and incoherence.

Sleep was impossible and I more or less passed out until the pain medication wore off. As time progressed, my understanding of the surgeon's prognosis rang true. My tolerance to the pain medications was rendering them less and less effective at postponing my having to hold my authentic self – post injury. If I am honest, I spent the first five years after my injury, trying to comprehend the change I had gone through.

The notion of never being the same was not a surprise. I had understood the surgeon's prognosis. Living that path of eroding uncertainty was terrifying.

> I felt as though no one could possibly understand the isolating nature of my suffering. I was separated from those I loved, and worse … my Self.

Only my son was able to love me unconditionally through my pain. Everyone else saw me as angry and bitter. In truth, I was vulnerable and loving, but the affect of so much pain presented as anger to all but a few sensitive souls. When my six –year-old son had to defend his dad to my own family, I knew my time was up. No more avoiding. No more false hope. I had to begin the process of fashioning my inner Self in order to bring my pain and suffering into a normative balance. Easier said than done, but absolutely necessary.

Over the last five years, I have spent one year initially going off all of my pain medications. I needed a baseline of who and how I was without a pharmaceutical lens. I spent a whole six months holding the full force of my new body. I gained a clear understanding of how changed I was the moment I hit the ground.

I did not regret keeping my foot – pain and all. As a mental health worker, I specialized in psychotic populations. I am poignantly aware of the isolation and suffering that is part of profound mental illness. Unlike many of my patients, I had an inner scaffolding from which I could reconfigure my newly emerging Self.

Most importantly, I had to love my pain. My pain was now a permanent part of who I am and who I was to become. I wanted my son to know a father who accepted adversity with dignity, not a man who ran from his pain.

The last four years have given rise to a human being I am grateful to be. I sleep very little (two to four hours) daily. My diet is now liquid only. I eat Soylent, an engineered food source. I am back on a minimal dosage of pain medication to balance everything.

> I know that this statement will sound strange,
> but if I could wave a magic wand and make my
> pain go away, I would not.

My perception these days is in each moment and no longer bound to time. My inner Self is orchestrated to manage my pain. In fact, I would go so far as to suggest that I have designed my Self around managing my pain.

I can only speak for myself, but the quality of life in relationship and existence has been a genuine gift. I believe that pain and suffering are part of the human condition – by design. How we humans hold the pain we experience, defines us.

With all that I have been through, I only wish I could communicate the gift pain brings to those who suffer with pain. For those who might doubt my sincerity, I am writing this paper seven days post-surgery. A consequence of my ankle pain is that my body is under tremendous stress. My dentist could no longer keep up with how quickly my teeth were eroding.

Seven days ago, I had every tooth in my head extracted (a ten hour surgery) and my jaw reshaped from years of pain clenching. I am in excruciating pain as I am writing these words. Yet, I am also grateful to be able to write such words.

Whether pain is by design, or we design around pain, one thing is constant – if you are a human being, you will experience pain and pain will experience you.

* * *

PART TWO:

The Outside View

To the Caregiver

By and large, (with some notable exceptions,) it is safe to assume that caregivers have the best of intentions. They want to deliver the best of care not only medically but also in terms of emotional support. Therefore, it is in the interest of maximizing their quality of care that the suggestions in this section are offered, not in the interest of attack or criticism. Sometimes it is helpful to know the ideal we are pursuing even if we can't be perfect in achieving it.

Think of the following questions as signposts on the road.

1. How is your energy?

If you let yourself absorb the information in Part One on a heart and gut level and are beginning to understand the internal world of a person in pain, this will make a dramatic difference in itself. Genuine empathy is *felt* in the room. It is a spirit of loving kindness that reaches into the hearts of those who suffer and lets us feel seen. It is altogether different from the forced cheerfulness of the caregiver who bursts in with an "everybody up for volleyball" kind of enthusiasm. With empathy, we feel *met* rather than blasted with another's presence.

> *I remember being woken up at six a.m. in hospital after three or four hours' sleep with a glaringly bright light in my eyes and a nurse announcing stridently: "It's time to take your blood pressure!" I silently wished I could punch her and then push her out the door. It is a nasty shock to the system to be woken up like that. It might even be seen as sadistic.*

Each one of us has an energy that we bring into the field. Being a therapist requires being attuned to this energy in ourselves as well as in the other. Emotions are contagious. Research on mirror neurons shows that we are activated by emotions in the other even when they are not outwardly expressed. Part of the work of caregiving is tuning into the impact of your presence on the other as well as theirs on you.

Like therapists, people in pain tend to be acutely sensitive to the energy of each person who enters their space and either soothes or agitates them. Yet too often caregivers seem to be oblivious to the impact they have. Some come in with a cold robotic professionalism, others with a dark gloomy cloud over their heads, and still others with a bustling impatience to do what they came for and be done with you. Perhaps they are carrying problems on the ward or in their personal lives that have nothing to do with you. They are human beings after all. Nonetheless, the bottom line is the care of the patient. It must be recognized that it can have a decidedly negative impact on the vulnerable patient to be treated in these ways.

One of the nurses had a cold sullen expression. She handled me roughly and she never smiled. This was at a time when I was at my worst. I was stretched to the limit just dealing with my own condition. I found myself dreading her appearance at the door. I felt myself cringing when she came near my bed. To make matters worse, that week she was working three days in a row. The prospect of three days with her as my nurse raised feelings of dread in me.

My son and I decided as an experiment to see if we could cheer her up. That would be a win-win for both sides. We found out that she really liked ice cream but hadn't had any in a very long time. My son went to Coldstone Creamery and got some fancy ice cream for her. She seemed pleased and was softer after that. I'd vote for ice cream for all the nurses if it would help them put aside their problems for the sake of patients who may already have more than they can handle dealing with their own pain.

Being present with another so that you are focused on them and fully engaged in listening and responding to their state of mind at the moment is a skill. It is a skill that is part of our training as therapists and is needed by medical practitioners as well. It means putting aside your personal issues and responding only within the context of the patient. Ultimately, it implies a centeredness and self-assurance that may be more of a constant striving than an accomplished goal. However, it is what we are there to do as caregivers. It is an essential part of the job.

If it is required by the job and difficult to do, there is a need for education and training. Possibilities might include workshops, group or individual communication sessions, feedback about the caregiver's impact, supervision and maybe even (last but not least) therapy. This may sound idealistic and impractical. However, if hospitals and insurance companies came to see that the energy with which we care for patients has a direct relation to their healing and, specifically, the length of time they spend in hospital, it might appear cost-effective to invest in training of this sort.

2. How is your touch?

Touch is an element that is often overlooked or minimized. Yet it plays a crucial role in the health and well-being of each of us.

From the beginning, infants require touching and holding as much as they require food, water, and warmth. The needs for emotional and physical closeness are not a luxury but occupy a position on a par with basic physiological needs. The research of French psychologist René Spitz[13] during the Second World War revolutionized psychology by establishing this point. War-orphaned infants who were fed, clothed and cared for on a physical level nonetheless sickened and even died because they were not rocked and held by the beleaguered staff of the orphanage. We can never again conceptualize human beings as purely physical creatures. We need to be touched and held to survive, not to mention, to thrive.

My son David spent all sixteen days in the hospital with me, mostly lying beside me on the bed. Since the time my sons were little, I always had a bedtime ritual of lying beside each one in turn, reading, singing or playing games every night before they went to sleep. I have always regarded it as a very important and meaningful ritual. Even now that they are adults, we often have our deep conversations lying side by side on the bed. It is a way of bonding that combines physical and emotional closeness in a powerful healing way.

One day as we cuddled together on the bed, the head-nurse on the floor marched in and demanded that David get up and sit in the chair. "You can't be there!" she declared with muted outrage, implying that we were doing something blatantly wrong. My son quietly and calmly replied: "This is healing for my mom and it makes her feel better so I'm not moving." "You're refusing to move?" the nurse repeated, obviously in shock that her order was not being immediately obeyed. "Well, then," she said with a tone of dark foreboding, "you'll have to talk with the supervisor!" "Fine," we both answered at the same time.

---

[13] Spitz, René, *The First Year of Life*, International Universities Press, New York, 1965 quoted in Aarons, Rachel B.: *Journey to Home: Quintessential Therapy and Beyond*, Journey Press, Santa Barbara, 2009, pp. 16 - 17.

The supervisor showed up the next day to investigate our questionable behavior. We reiterated our truth. It was healing and it did help me to have him close beside me. She looked at us both lying there smiling at her and, to her credit, she said "okay" and went away. We were never bothered about it again.

Loving touch is healing. On two conditions. One, the patient welcomes the touch and two, the touch is genuinely loving.

In the first case, there are some of us who are simply not open to receiving a loving touch. Permission needs to be given and sometimes it is withheld.

Just as I came to write this section, I happened on an interview with Virginia Satir, one of the pioneers of family therapy and an important teacher of mine. The interviewer was wondering how it was that Virginia was able to get people whom other therapists might consider unbudgeable to make changes in their lives. Virginia replied:

"I had an experience once that taught me a lot about how to lead people to scary places. I wanted to descend into a cave but was very frightened. My friend said, "I'll carry the light. If you give me your hand and allow me to lead the way, then maybe we can go down together." Unless he had been willing to give me his hand and unless the hand felt trustworthy, I would not have gone."[14]

Hands may not feel trustworthy, according to Virginia, if your hand is sending "dominating messages."[15] The patient may feel like an object to be moved around and manipulated rather than as a person with thoughts and feelings.[16] It is easy

---

[14] Simon, Richard, *Reaching out to life: An Interview with Virginia Satir,* PsychotherapyNetworker.org/free-reports/, November 2014, pp. 2 – 3.

[15] *Ibid.*, p. 3.

[16] The distinction I am making is reminiscent of Buber's distinction between I-It and I-Thou relationships. cf. Buber, Martin, *I and Thou,* Charles Scribner's Sons, New York, 1958.

to understand how the system of medical procedures repeated at regular intervals, day and night, day after day, can deaden the patient/caregiver relationship on both sides. Reaching out a hand is an offer of connection. We may need to hold hands to break through the deadness and feel each other's presence. It is a relief to have a companion on the road.

> *I think my doctor would have been a hit with Virginia Satir. He always reached out to hold my hand. He had enormous warm hands that enveloped me in warmth and safety. What I remembered most vividly about him from the outset were his amazing hands.*

3. How much do you share?

Doctors are not omniscient and they make mistakes. It can happen. They may or may not take responsibility for their errors in judgment or knowledge. Sometimes it turns out that the misinformation they give can have lifelong consequences as we learn in the following story.

My Unique Son: Donna Nelson

At fourteen, I started suffering from severe abdominal pain. It hurt to stand up straight and it hurt to wear clothes. I couldn't read a page and tell you the contents. The doctors could not figure out what was wrong so I had nerve blocks every six to eight weeks and was given bottles of Darvon Compound-65 so I could function. It was suggested that I needed a change. Perhaps if I was away from home, I would feel better. I went to Europe with a prescription and instructions on nerve blocks, just in case. Although it was a chaperoned tour, the leaders did not accompany me to the hospitals in either country we visited, including the one where I did not speak the language. I remember feeling very alone, riding buses to the hospitals that said they would give me a nerve block. I was only fourteen years old and in pain when I took that trip.

My high school years were a blur of pain and pills. The summer between high school and college, I met my future husband. A year later, miraculously, I was free of pain. I thought it was because I was so happy – I had heard for so long that they could find no physical cause for my agony. Twelve years later, it turned out that I had endometriosis, and had had it for fifteen years. It is rare for someone to have that condition at such a young age. It was going on birth control pills that ended my discomfort.

I had gone off birth control to get pregnant. It was all planned out. Go off the pill in the spring, get pregnant in August, September or October, and have our first child the next spring. What I had not counted on was the pain returning. In August I had a laparoscopy and was told I would not be able to get pregnant. I was put on Danocrine and the doctor warned that I must not get pregnant on the drug or I could have the equivalent of a thalidomide baby.

I returned to the doctor in September complaining about the heavy bleeding I was experiencing. At the time, I was teaching Kindergarten wearing two tampons and a pad. There were many times I just made it out the door before blood was all over the classroom floor. It got so bad that some days I went through several changes of clothes. The doctor said that break-through bleeding was common on this drug. This seemed more like hemorrhaging to me. The blood clots were up to six inches in diameter. Hot flashes were another side effect. I was taking a night class when I got a particularly long one. I thought if I stayed quiet and did not draw any attention to myself that no one would notice. I was wrong. The instructor noticed how red I was and came over to fan me. I was the only woman in the class and I was very embarrassed.

In October, I called the doctor's office again. They said they didn't need to see me and that what I was experiencing were normal side effects. A colleague at school insisted that I go back in. She had seen the pools of blood and was concerned.

My appointment was for 3:00 on a Friday afternoon. The doctor told me I was pregnant. I knew that if I was pregnant, I had to be at least twelve weeks into the pregnancy. They argued that this was not possible and sent me downstairs for an ultrasound and blood work. It took quite a while and it was just after 5:00 when I returned. The receptionist told me I was so late she thought I had left. I explained that it was the ultrasound and lab work that had taken so long. Then she turned off all the lights in the waiting room and left me sitting in the dark. This was an apt metaphor for the state I was in.

Some time later, the nurse noticed me and brought me back into an examining room. Test results showed that I was twelve weeks pregnant. This meant that I had been two weeks pregnant when I had the laparoscopy and was told I could not get pregnant. I had taken the drug for ten weeks! They said that my baby would have shortened limbs and characteristics of both sexes. An abortion was scheduled for the following Friday.

My husband was out of town for the weekend. My parents were in court that week going through a very messy divorce. I was at a loss as to what to do. I went to the mall and walked around the children's clothing store, thinking and praying. When I got home, there was a box of Godiva chocolates in the mail. I sat sobbing and ate the whole pound, except the two coffee chocolates.

My mother was thrilled to be a grandmother of my brother's six-month-old boy and my sister's two-month-old girl. It was not the time to tell her about the new grandchild she might have. Suffice it to say, it was a very long weekend.

On Monday, I was surprised to be congratulated on being pregnant. A parent of one of my students had a cousin who worked in the lab. All the parents waiting to pick up their children knew about the pregnancy before I had told my mother, or even decided what to do.

My father is a doctor. I called him and asked him to meet me in a city half way between the places where we each lived. It made sense to me that if we both drove one and a half hours to meet, it would be easier than one of us driving three hours. He told me he didn't like to drive at night and didn't want to meet. He did get me an appointment for a second opinion, however.

At my appointment, I found out that they could tell from the ultrasound that my baby did not have shortened limbs. The doctor did some research and reported that if I had a boy, there would not be any sexual deformities because I was taking a male hormone. If I had a girl, there could be deformities; however, they would require only simple surgery to repair. This baby was wanted and loved. I decided against the abortion. I also decided not to return to the first doctor.

The pregnancy was not ideal. My baby suffered from intrauterine growth retardation. He was born at thirty-two weeks weighing only three pounds. It was two and a half months until he was big enough to nurse. At seven months, he had a near-miss SIDS and stopped breathing. At a year, he weighed twelve pounds, did not move, and made no sounds. Walking did not happen until age two and a half. Walking on grass or uneven ground until age four and a half. He had years of physical, occupational, and speech therapy.

No one would say that his problems were caused by the drug I had taken. Brain scans showed holes where his brain did not grow in utero. Some of his diagnoses are: Attention Deficit Disorder, dyscalculia (math dyslexia), disgraphia (writing problems), an Auditory Processing Disorder, a hearing loss so unique the specialists thought he had a brain tumor, bladder problems, poor gross motor skills, no fine motor skills, scoliosis, Growth Hormone Deficiency, Pervasive Developmental Disorder NOS, and Asperger's Syndrome. One leg is longer from the ankle to the knee and the other is longer from the knee to the hip. This gives him an unusual gait. I have lost count of the specialists we have taken him to. The one thing that has been agreed upon is that he is unique and complicated.

My son has made me a much better teacher. I understand about a variety of learning disabilities because he has so many of them. Currently he is thirty years old chronologically and twelve years old emotionally. Testing has shown he scores from the 98th percentile in visual discrimination, and to the 2nd percentile in math. He can seem totally brilliant and unbelievably dense all in the period of five minutes. He is kind, caring and likes to help others. He is also impulsive, messy, and gullible. He will never be independent. He has brought me pain, heartache, and joy.

My husband died suddenly six years ago. He told me if we had it to do over again, he would have chosen the abortion. He always mourned the child he wished we had. For myself, I wish I had not seen the first OB GYN, gone to that clinic, or taken the Danocrine. I wish things had been easier for my son. Life has been difficult. However, I do not regret my decision to keep my son.

* * *

It is said that information is power. However, this is tricky in reference to the medical world.

In their need-to-know, patients occupy places on a continuum somewhere between two opposite extremes. The more traditional approach is to follow your doctor's advice without question. The doctor is perceived as the expert who knows what he or she is doing. Your job is to trust their expertise without needing much in the way of explanation. It may even feel disrespectful to ask a lot of questions, as if you were questioning the authority of the doctor to prescribe. At this end of the continuum, the patient role is a fundamentally a passive one.

In recent years, more emphasis has been placed on patient responsibility for our own care. We need to gain an understanding of our own condition, hunt down resources that summarize what is known in the field, and research treatment options so that we can make a responsible decision about the medical route we will follow. The patient role at this end of the continuum is an engaged and proactive one.

Hence, doctors and nurses face a diversity of patient needs when it comes to the sharing of information. Some patients may want to know more, some less. At the same time, it is, I would argue, the responsibility of medical providers to offer all the relevant information they have to those patients who are open to receiving it. And they need to offer it well enough in advance that patients who prefer to make their own decisions have the opportunity to do so. This is not always what happens.

I was lying on a hospital bed already sedated at the precise time booked for my surgery when my surgeon came in to tell me that I needed to decide if I would have two additional procedures during the surgery, one to be performed by an anaestheologist and one by a urologist. These two doctors, neither of whom I had met before, filed in one after the other to discuss my decisions and obtain my consent. I was in no position to decide anything at that time. The insertion of a central line came across to me as opening up a hole in my neck to draw out blood and all I could think of were vampire movies. In regard to the second procedure, I never had (or, at least, never retained) any understanding of what the urology stint was for. I am the type of person who likes a lot of information and needs time to process the information, including running it by other people in order to come to a decision myself. Obviously, this was not possible under the circumstances. Fortunately, in my case, it was not critical to the surgery that the consent I gave was not informed consent. However, it was disturbing to me to be put in this position just before I was going into surgery. I don't think it was helpful either.

Would my client with cancer have risked the back surgery had she known that it could result in her being paralyzed?

At the very same time as I was in hospital for the sixteen days, my older son, Kieran, had been going through surgery in another country. However, it turned out that his wound was not healing as was hoped. The surgeon proposed a second surgery, assuring him that the wound would heal quickly and successfully if he went ahead.

Unfortunately, the second surgery was not successful. Kieran had a much larger incision and eighty percent of his stitches did not adhere. He felt that he was thrown back three months and was doing worse than before the latest surgery. He was understandably angry and upset. When Kieran confronted the issue, the surgeon told him that it was a risky procedure that often didn't work. Although the doctor never provided statistics, it was clear that, had my son known of the risk, he would not have gone forward with the surgery. Withholding that information was wrong. The patient has a right to know.

In the cancer arena, each patient develops and works with a team of doctors. The idea is that they are all connected with one another and, at the same time, connected with you.

In principle, the team approach is based on the assumption that all the members are focused on a common goal – your healing. Information is shared. You are even assigned a "patient navigator" whose role is to help you move through the system as seamlessly as possible and to ensure that all your questions are answered. I would advocate for the team approach in every area of medicine not only between doctors but also between your doctors and you.

As Virginia Satir says, "When people come to see me, I don't ask them if they want to change. I just assume they do. I don't tell them what's wrong with them or what they ought to do. I just offer my hand literally and metaphorically… I say, 'Where do you want to go?'…Being asked that question shocks many people. They cannot believe that anybody really wants to know the direction in which they want to go… As a therapist, I am a companion. I try to help people to tune into their own wisdom."[17] Would that our doctors and nurses, friends and family, were always companions of this sort.

> *As an example, my doctor (the one with the amazing hands) spelled out exactly what he was thinking, the assumptions underlying his hypotheses, and the pros and cons of the choices confronting me. He allowed it to be **my** decision in the full meaning of the word. I had a sense of ownership of what would follow. Since I would be the one suffering the consequences, it seems right that I should take responsibility for the decision. He was not pushing me. We were part of a team.*

4. Perils of hospital life

A hospital stay is not like a stay at the Four Seasons. Or even a stay at the Best Western. No matter how newly decorated and

---

[17] Simon, Richard, *Reaching out to Life: An Interview with Virginia Satir*, p. 3.

well appointed the hospital, it is not like a hotel stay at all. It is a place you go to treat an illness. Hopefully it is a place of healing but, of necessity, it has features that are not at all healing. You will have to work with it to maximize the benefits and minimize the deficits.

As the nurses often repeat, the hospital is not a place to go for sleep. Getting any decent sleep in a hospital is a formidable challenge.

> *The first night when I was, unexpectedly, admitted into hospital, I was sent to the ICU. It was organized as a circle of beds separated by curtains and arranged around a central nurses' station. The idea, I presume, was that you could be supervised at all hours of the day or night. As a result, I had very little privacy. The curtains had a top section with no material so the light shone right in my eyes. The nurses conducted their business in their normal voices so there was talking all the time. I could also hear visitors in the next cubicles as if they were inside mine. Nurses kept checking on my vital signs at frequent intervals. People were coming in and out all the time since emergencies do not adhere to a regular schedule. It becomes clear that if you going to get any sleep at all, you will have to find a way to go below the noise or rise above it. I was very relieved to be transferred to a single hospital room the next day.*

Patients are generally given hospital gowns to wear. They are practical and convenient. However, after a few days of padding around in a hospital gown, you may begin to feel more like an inmate in a prison than the person you were a few days before. A nice robe from home can be of some help in embellishing the otherwise depressing patient uniform. But I quickly discovered that getting dressed in my street clothes and putting on make-up was a jump-start to my sense of self.

As soon as I was able, I declared my basic right to a shower on a daily basis. My little ritual of showering, dressing and putting on make-up, although it was a frustratingly lengthy process, was well worth the effort. I felt so much better when I was walking around looking like a normal person. There is more than enough in the experience of being a patient that is an assault on your dignity as you are poked and prodded and examined inside and out. It may not always be healthy to fully embrace the patient role. Thus it was disconcerting, even discouraging, to be told that, apparently, I was the only one on the floor who did this.

A hospital room can be a very small space. The longer you are there, the more the room seems to constrict in space. This is within the context of a world that, as we have seen above, is already shrinking as you become more and more preoccupied with illness and pain. The more exclusively you focus on pain, the more pain you feel. So it becomes imperative for your healing that you find ways to expand the space you occupy in any way you can.

Depending on your condition, part of your therapy may be walking the halls. Doing so reminds you that there are other people, coming and going, other worlds beside the one you are in most of the time. Seeing people in street clothes in the front lobby or in the cafeteria wakes you up to the containment of the hospital world and highlights the fact that there is another reality out there that you hope to rejoin one day soon. Even if walking is not an option, it helps to bring in reminders of the world you call home. These could be photos, objects of art, flowers, or comfort objects like stuffed animals. For me, the most transformative setting was getting outside where the air was fresh and something was growing and flowering,

Again, unlike most of the patients on my floor, I took full advantage of the night hours to walk the halls with my son. There were less people around and we appreciated

the sense of privacy it gave us. What turned out to be the most beneficial aspect of the hospital ward were the outside patios that we hung out on both by day and by night. During the day, I entertained visiting friends on the patio. At night, even in the dark, we sat out and talked. The shadows of trees, the moonlight, the hint of nature beyond the walls of the building restored a feeling of connection to the world. It seemed possible - out there - that I would eventually get out of that place. It was a source of hope.

In general, there *is* reason for hope. Hundreds of thousands of patients pass in and out of hospitals on a daily basis. Most of them are success stories. Thanks to the expertise of the hospital staff, most patients are able to recover from their illnesses and move on. Most of their experiences are positive.

However, I want to take a look at two exceptions, exemplified by two different patient stories. The most frightening aspect of the first story is how it leads us to wonder how many similar examples may be occurring on a regular basis in hospitals across the nation.

Drama in the Emergency Room: Anne's Story

It all began one day when a fall from three feet brought my left buttock and cement together, knocking the air out of me. I was standing on a stepstool washing my car when my flip flop turned over and I lost my balance. Fortunately, I suffered no broken bones. I was seventy years old at the time so that was a big relief.

As the weeks passed, pain from an irreversible degenerative disease of the spine steadily increased and found new areas of my body in which to reek havoc.

Finally, on a holiday weekend, the severe pain forced me to visit the Emergency Room seeking relief. It was extremely busy that day so they were setting up beds in the hallways. At first, they placed me in a room where I could overhear a woman reporting black patches on her skin. The nurses seemed seriously concerned and I was happy when they moved me into the hallway.

I had mentioned in front of an intern that I wished my daughter were there to act as an advocate for me. Then this woman appeared, announcing: "My name is Donna." She was about to administer an injection for me but she was not dressed in nursing attire. Was she supposed to be my advocate?

Since I had fallen on my left side, I asked her to give me the shot on the right side. She was very annoyed by this request and kicked the bed away from the wall to reach my other side. Then she started shouting: "Lower! Lower!" to get my pants pulled farther down. It was very difficult and painful for me to move. She said: "You bother me!" and I did not react. Then she remarked with disdain: "It could not have been very high," referring to the height I fell from. Why would she say something like that to me? I was obviously suffering and it felt like she just dismissed my pain.

The doctor was unable to bring up my previous MRI on their computer so they ordered an X-ray and a scan of my spine. Both results were normal, the doctor said.

I had to wait a long time for the results of the MRI. The doctor showed surprise in his voice when he reported to me: "You really *do* have a cyst on your spine!" Did he think I was feigning pain? I was relieved that they finally had found a reason to believe my pain was real. Finally some credibility!

Donna returned to organize my discharge and said with a tone of extreme irritation: "I will call in your prescriptions if and when I get time." I was amazed that she continued in her attitude of contempt even when it was evident that I had a serious pain condition.

It was her job to call a taxicab for me. I passed her a card and she sneered at it as if I was lying. I turned it over to show her the taxicab number on the reverse side. The thought crossed my mind:"Does she think I am calling my drug dealer?" That's how outrageous her attitude was.

The following week I went to my neurologist and he wondered why they had not identified the problem in the first two tests. Then I found out I actually had not one but two cysts in the lumbar region caused by leaking spinal fluid. That was the source of my severe pain. By then, I was fortunate to be able to get the first of several epidurals and finally some relief from the pain.

The whole experience in the Emergency Room was shocking, with an air of the surreal. It has stayed with me ever since. I felt treated like a criminal who was there just to get pain medication, despite the fact that I already had my own pain medication with me. I just needed to understand what was wrong with my body. Instead, I felt attacked and disbelieved. Was this because they regarded me as a patient of advanced age who could not be counted on to report reliably? Was this elder abuse as one of my internists suggested? I am still in a quandary about this more than two years later.

When a person goes to the Emergency unit, they are generally frightened, vulnerable and distressed. On top of dealing with the acute situation that brought them there, they may also have to deal with rude and deprecating treatment from the staff. How can we justify an attitude on the part of the hospital professionals that makes a patient feel disrespected and disbelieved?

My neurologist commented:"This is how you will find it in ER's across the United States." If this is true, it is a sad comment on the state of care for patients who go for help to the Emergency Room.

* * *

The second story is nothing less than a horror story. It moves us to take action to ensure that similar examples will never recur anytime or anywhere.

A Medication Nightmare: Mary-Grace's Story

PAIN

This silent awful journey I must go forth alone.
Daggers fly toward my pureness, but I stay
in prayer pose, and my battle has just begun.
Bringing peace of mind to others is my job
right now. Just adding a smile, I await
the great journey that waits for my arrival.
Flames engulf my breath, my innocence.
And I stay hoping that the fiery orange inferno
is no more than an illusion of my pain.
My eyes roll back and this vile sensation takes
its course.
I am waiting for my release from this …
BUT, I asked for a price and this is what I pay?

~Mary-Grace Langhorne

It all started with a cough. Mary-Grace was put on antibiotics and she developed a gag reflex. She had an allergic reaction to the codeine she was given and could not eat or drink. She was on IV when she was admitted to the hospital the first time. A pediatric psychiatrist at Santa Barbara Cottage Hospital suspected she had PANDAS and suggested she be referred to U.C.L.A. This was January of 2013. She was eleven years old at the time.

PANDAS or Pediatric Autoimmune Neuropsychiatric Disorder is associated with streptococcal infections. "The term is used to describe a subset of children who have Obsessive Compulsive Disorder and/or tic disorders such as Tourette Syndrome, and in whom symptoms worsen following strep infections such as "Strep Throat" and Scarlet Fever. The children usually have dramatic 'overnight' onset of symptoms, including motor or vocal tics, obsessions, and/or compulsions. In addition to these symptoms, children may also become moody, irritable or show concerns about separating from parents or loved ones. The abrupt onset is generally preceded by a Strep throat infection."[18] In Mary-Grace's case, the strep infection was missing so the provisional diagnosis was PANDA.

Mary-Grace's mother told me they were excited to go to U.C.L.A. in the hope and expectation that they would receive help for their daughter. Nothing could be farther from the truth.

At the recommendation of a psychology intern, Mary-Grace was administered Haloperidol (brand name Haldol) intravenously, rather than intramuscularly as is usually recommended and without the Benadryl which normally accompanies it. She had an extreme reaction. Her temperature spiked, her blood pressure and her pulse escalated and

---

[18] The National Institute of Mental Health, www.nimh.nih.gov/health/publications/pandas/index.shtml

she developed tachycardia. "She almost died," Mary-Grace's mother said.

Mary-Grace described her experience with Haldol in these words:

"They tried to give it to me by mouth but my gag reflex went crazy so they used an IV. I went into hysteria, had hallucinations, and started having a seizure. They left the room."

A total of four doses were administered by IV before the order was cancelled. Rather than reevaluating this course of medication in the light of the patient's reactions, they continued to give her additional doses that were three to five times stronger than usual due to the fact that they were given intravenously.

After the 3rd injection of Haldol," Mary-Grace reported, "I started frothing at the mouth. I felt like my brain was melting. I was so hot it was like being in hell." For these extreme temperatures and involuntary muscle spasms, they started injecting Dantrolene and it paralyzed her. Within twenty-four hours, her mother confirmed, Mary-Grace could no longer walk.

"The fourth injection I remember so well," Mary-Grace continued. "I took a walk in the hall with my mom and I fell backward. My back arched and my arms twisted back. I couldn't breathe and I blacked out. I woke up to arm cuffs and an EEG."

They kept administering Dantrolene and her reactions were horrific. "I felt as if I had lava in my brain and beetles on my face. When I had to throw up, I aspirated and couldn't breathe. They were suctioning my lungs. It felt like at least a liter of froth came out of my mouth and my pupils were as big as sharks. My hands were seizing and my neck twisted back. My back went out on me and I was limp as a noodle. I was unable to talk. A church man was praying for me. It was like an exorcism."

Unfortunately this "exorcism" was not healing. A few days later when she was able to talk, Mary-Grace asked her parents what had happened. "They told me I did not have Tourette's but a Conversion Disorder. They did not explain what that meant, except to say it was 'psychogenic'." No explanation of Conversion Disorder was given by U.C.LA. to her parents either. Although hospital protocol was to call Child Protective Services in the event of a diagnosis of Conversion Disorder because of the possibility of child abuse, no report was made at that time. Instead, she was transferred to Children's Hospital.

A psychologist at Children's Hospital gave the explanation the family was looking for. It was all in her head and she could control it, they were told. "I refused to believe this," Mary-Grace said, "and I told the psychologist that I had an adverse reaction to the medication. I told my parents, my friends, the doctors and anybody who would listen."

Evidently the staff at Children's Hospital believed the U.C.L.A. diagnosis and not the patient. The treatment she received was based on the assumption that Mary-Grace was in conscious control of her symptoms and simply refused to cooperate. Because they believed she could walk, compulsory physical therapy for three to four hours every day was required. They refused to give her a wheel chair or a walker. They would let her fall and would not help her up. Her mother believes that trying to walk on partially paralyzed limbs and legs injured her and made her recovery longer. They made her sleep on a mat on the linoleum floor in her hospital room because they would not help her climb into her bed. She had to dress herself on the ground by crawling to the closet. They made her crawl on hands and knees in the hallways and crawl her way up the stairs, refusing to assist her when she fell hard on her tailbone multiple times and was crying in pain. They made her stand in a standing box for one to two hours straight and they tried to force her to get up in a group exercise. "I kept trying but I kept falling down. Other kids got breaks but not me. Other kids could have their parents there, but they wouldn't let my mom be there with me."

The policy of the hospital was that parents could stay with their children twenty-four hours a day. However, in Mary-Grace's case, it was limited to *three* hours a day. Mary-Grace was very attached to her mother and this was especially hard on her. She hated sleeping alone because she shared a room with her sisters at home. Although she requested a double room, she was given a single. They wouldn't allow her to go into her room during the day. She had to stay in the common area where the nurse's station was located. They took away the TV and the telephone as "a no-electronics protocol for Conversion Disorder." She hid her iPod but they found it and removed it too. When she hit her head on the toilet, the nurse who was initially nice to her read her chart and thought she was lying. So she took away the ice bag that had been given to soothe her pain. This hospital stay was nothing short of torture.

After three weeks of this ordeal, Mary-Grace's mother removed her from Children's Hospital when they refused to reevaluate her treatment regimen. She was taken home and remained there until the damage to her foot began to escalate. It developed into chronic regional pain disorder. At that point, she was admitted into Northridge Hospital in the pediatric intensive care unit.

The experience at Northridge turned out to be more of the same. After being admitted for chronic regional pain disorder and dystonia, they tried to force her to go back to U.C.L.A. despite their knowledge of how she had suffered from U.C.L.A.'s mismanagement of her medications.

The medical staff at Northridge insisted that she could eat when food would block her oesophyagus and come back up.

Her doctor would only allow her to have medications by swallowing and she would aspirate every time. They actually went so far as to contact Child Protective Services in an attempt to remove parental rights so they could force her to return to U.C.L.A., claiming that her parents were not holding her best interests. Child Protective Services of Santa Barbara refused to act upon the hospital's complaint so they contacted Child Protective Services of Los Angeles. Her parents got a lawyer and again CPS sided with the parents against the hospital. Clearly, this was not a safe place for their daughter so her parents took action. They hired a private ambulance and private doctors and, as Mary-Grace described it, in a drama like Mission Impossible, they managed to rescue her from Northridge Hospital.

Her parents set up a triage center at their home with doctors and registered nurses around the clock while they attempted to get Mary-Grace to Stanford Children's Hospital. After ten weeks of suffering chronic regional pain disorder, post-traumatic stress disorder, and dystonia, she finally was medivac'd by jet to Stanford Hospital. There she endured one more week of much the same kind of treatment. Since her feet would straighten out under anesthesia, the doctor at Stanford concluded it was under her control and called it a "psychogenic dystonia." Just like the other three hospitals, he disregarded the report of the foot doctor about the damage to her feet and persisted in the belief that it was all in her head.

Why would a hospital treat a patient this way? Why would *four* major hospitals persist in the same conviction despite all contrary evidence? Each read the diagnosis of the previous one and failed to question it. They supported each other in a manner reminiscent of an "old boys' network." At the source was a mistake in the administration of medication that nobody wanted to take responsibility for. Instead of accepting the blame, they passed it along to the patient, in this case an eleven-year-old girl, and felt justified in treating her in a extraordinarily inhumane way. [19]

Mary-Grace is now thirteen years old and still working to recover from her ordeal. The misdiagnosis by U.C.L.A. has caused continued efforts by Mary Grace's parents and current health care practitioners to remedy this situation and, in essence, "un-ring the bell of misdiagnosis."

* * *

Is this an aberration? A one time case of arrogance gone wild? Lamentably, the treatment of patients with fibromyalgia, chronic fatigue syndrome, and myalgic encephalomyelitis (ME) show marked commonalities with Mary-Grace's case. These are also conditions that are viewed not as a medical illness but as a psychiatric one.

5. Attitudes toward Psychosomatic Illness

The film "Voices from the Shadows" which addresses the problem of ME begins with the words: "If we become seriously ill, we all expect to be treated with compassion and helped to regain our health. We don't expect to be disbelieved, blamed for being ill or dismissed by the medical profession."[20]

To understand the symptoms of ME, picture ME patients lying in darkened rooms with blind folds over their eyes to

---

[19] Conversion Disorder is described as: "One or more symptoms or deficits affecting voluntary motor or sensory function that suggest a neurological or other general medical condition...The symptom or deficit cannot, after appropriate investigation, be fully explained by a general medical condition, or by the direct effects of a substance, or as a culturally sanctioned behavior or experience." Diagnostic Criteria From DSM-IV, American Psychiatric Association, Washington, DC, 1994, pp. 221-22. It might be argued that the symptoms or deficits in this case can, in fact, be attributed to the direct effects of a substance – namely Haldol.

[20] *Voices From the Shadows*, https://vimeo.com/on demand.

protect them from light and ear phones (turned off) on their ears to protect them from sound, racked with pain, unable to care for themselves, often for years on end. Patients with ME and their caregivers described experiences that hauntingly echo what Mary-Grace had to say.

- My suffering was belittled and undermined;
- I was met with disbelief and hostility;
- I was made to feel like a criminal doing something wrong;
- I was treated differently from other patients;
- She was told she was making it up; that her illness was in her mind;
- She was dragged around the corridor and not allowed to have a wheelchair because they said she could walk;
- She was forced to do graded exercise although evidence showed that such exercises made the condition worse;
- At her worst, she was completely paralyzed;
- She couldn't swallow so had to be tube fed;
- Her mother was banned from entering the ward other than specific hours;
- Children were threatened with removal from their families and placement in foster care;
- There was abuse at the hands of medical professionals;

The medical establishment would not believe these patients had a debilitating medical illness and treated them as malingerers.

When an illness is treated as a psychiatric condition rather than a medical one as is the case for patients with ME and as it was with Mary-Grace, the patient suffers more than just severe physical pain. They suffer what can only be regarded as severe emotional pain at the hands of those they turn to for help – the medical profession.

We have entered the realm of what is known as *psychosomatic illness*. As in the case of suicide, this domain is remarkably complex, complicated, and highly controversial. To do it justice is well beyond the scope of this book. However, I will begin with a story by a woman who has had fibromyalgia and chronic fatigue since early childhood and now leads a fibromyalgia and chronic fatigue support group at Sansum Clinic in Santa Barbara.

* * *

Pain: Is it Psychosomatic?: Bonnie Scot

Extreme pain has been a part of my life since the age of four. After an auto accident and surgery, everything changed. My once-healthy and active child's body no longer worked. The simplest activities became pain-filled. Energy was unpredictable. Debilitating nausea would come and go. Bowel and bladder function diminished. Hard lumps formed in muscles that often cramped and went into spasm. Sensitivity to light and noise increased. Skin hurt, even hair hurt to be moved. Confusingly, all symptoms were intermittent and unpredictable, except for a constant whole body ache, which remained and worsened over time.

For many years, doctors thought I was pretending or making it all up, a child with an imagination that was too vivid and focused on illness rather than health. Some suggested I complained to garner attention, that I was insecure or manipulative. Some thought I was simply neurotic, bringing emotional upset down from the head and into the body. Some thought I had discovered a way to intentionally make my body appear sick.

There were times when, for months, I would feel as if the flu had come on and wouldn't go away, with chills and low-grade fever, constant sore throat and swollen glands, and always incredible aching. Even the feel of clothing or touching the metal of a door handle caused pain.

Coupled with the pain were periods of cognitive challenge. There were times when the simplest memories were lost, like forgetting the multiplication tables, how to wash dishes, or find my way home from the neighborhood grocery store. When feeling well, I built strength by dancing and other motor activities, but even when physically strong, there were times when muscles wouldn't work in coordinated ways. Walking became jerky, and weakness made any activity a challenge. If I did engage in a strenuous activity like horseback riding, I might be totally exhausted and in extreme pain for days after, unable to do anything. Fear of causing more pain inhibited choices.

The idea that nothing was physically wrong and that all the challenges were psychological or neurotic, became a recurring theme. Over and over I was told that these symptoms were mine alone, that no one else was affected in these difficult ways. I felt attacked and betrayed by my unreliable body and by the doctors trying to convince me it was my fault. Try as I might, nothing could make my body better.

One of the most hurtful aspects of living with fibromyalgia and chronic fatigue syndrome is being judged and criticized by people who do not understand the cognitive and physical challenges. Once school started, teachers described me as shy, stupid, lazy, or self-centered because at times I was unable to remember lessons or participate in activities. Some believed the problems were pretense and not real at all.

In 1998, while participating in a university pain study, a rheumatologist diagnosed these many symptoms as fibromyalgia and chronic fatigue syndrome. During a simple, five-minute exam he pressed gently on precise locations on my body and elicited tremendous pain. Pressing other locations caused no pain at all. With a huge sense of relief, I believed that knowing the cause of my pain would bring recommendations for a treatment or cure. Nothing was further from the truth. Naming the illness only seemed to give more ammunition for attack by believers in psychosomatic illness.

As part of the university study, participation in an education program using Cognitive Behavioral Therapy was required. I was hopeful, expecting to learn about ways to improve my physical experience. Instead, for months, a therapist insisted there was no pain, that imagination or a neurosis created the sense of pain; that in fact, I was psychologically making myself sick. This therapist was often rude, shouted, insulted, pressured for confession to these shortcomings. I finally left the program in fear and disgust, unwilling to pay for services that were abusive and that did not help to treat the source of pain.

This type of mistreatment continued with doctors in other specialties. For instance, after a cursory exam and x-rays, a knee specialist pressured for approval to perform surgical procedures while acknowledging that no pathology was apparent, nonetheless giving assurance that pain would disappear after the operations. What sense did that make?

Many years later, I learned of an experiment conducted on patients with knee pain. Some participants received surgery, some did not, although they all were anesthetized and cut, and told that a procedure had been done. One of the patients that did not receive the procedure experienced pain improvement thought to be attributable to what is known as the "placebo effect." Some doctors perceive this result as a justification for fake surgery, placing patients in a costly and potentially dangerous situation.

Such experiences were disheartening and frustrating. At times I simply refused to see doctors, being unwilling to face more abuse with no resolution of problems. My own search for information, however, yielded more positive results. A friend gave me a book written by the Arthritis Foundation in which it was suggested that 10% of severe arthritic pain was caused by food sensitivity, especially from the nightshades such as potatoes, tomatoes, and bell peppers. Detecting sensitivities can be difficult because it takes five to seven days for results to appear. Being a vegetarian at the time, my diet included these vegetables almost daily. Eliminating these foods over a period of months stopped the knee pain completely. Walking with a severe limp became walking with a smooth, regular gait, which became the ability to jog, and then run. Dancing became possible again.

Likewise, I discovered information about potential problems with gluten and sensitivities to other grains. Eliminating wheat, corn, oats, and barley from my diet almost completely eliminated skin pain and some digestive tract pain. Eliminating dairy also relieved some (though not all) bowel dysfunction and pain, especially the pain of burning mouth syndrome. Eliminating stimulants like coffee, caffeinated sodas, teas, and even chocolate reduced bladder pain and stopped repetitive urinary tract infections. These dietary choices brought about marked improvement in many of the symptoms, but in no way did they cure the disease.

Because I had been convinced as a child that the source of illness might somehow reside in my mind, psychiatry and psychotherapy seemed like logical healing pursuits. For years, practitioners in these "helping" professions were unable to change any aspect of the physical disease, and in many ways contributed to emotional suffering. In contrast, a skilled, compassionate psychotherapist specializing in depth psychology not only confirmed the physical reality of fibromyalgia and chronic fatigue syndrome, she offered constructive tools for managing the profound psychological challenges that accompany debilitating physical illness.

Interest in depth psychology prompted my research into the history of perceptions of physical illness interacting with the psyche. It is a strange history indeed. It is important to note that despite centuries of medical progress, patients with fibromyalgia and chronic fatigue syndrome may still be diagnosed as psychosomatic or hysterical.

In the late nineteenth century, Sigmund Freud published a theory that symptoms similar to those of FM/CFS were the result not of physical illness but of neurosis, whether called hysteria or neurasthenia, and attributed them instead to present or past sexual disturbances in the suffering patient.[21] The popularity of this theory has had a devastating impact on patients. Healthcare professionals untrained in psychology often feel free to judge a patient by this measure, having no knowledge of the patient's life, let alone their sexual history. Belief in this theory has precluded understanding of the physical and emotional devastation fibromyalgia, chronic fatigue syndrome, or any chronic pain condition can create.

Jean Martin Charcot, a contemporary of Freud, was a neurologist as well as psychiatrist, with interests in hysteria. His research focused on patients with a variety of painful, debilitating symptoms and he was ultimately able to medically identify diseases such as muscular sclerosis, Parkinson's disease, and amyotrophic lateral sclerosis (Lou Gehrig disease). Specific symptoms of these diseases lost their standing as hysterical and became medically legitimate. Fibromyalgia and

---

[21] Ellenberger Henri, *The Discovery of the Unconscious: The History and Evolution of Dynamic Psychiatry*, Basic Books, New York, 1981, p. 487.

chronic fatigue syndrome are only now in the same process of discovery.[22]

The history of medicine bears ample witness to this mistake. Seizure disorders such as epilepsy were early considered to be demonic possession. Later they were also thought to be contagious and acquired by people prone to developing an "epileptic character" which then, and often now, results in social stigma.[23]   Seizure disorders are neurological disorders having nothing to do with the patient's personality or psychological state.

Similarly, mercury vapor poisoning, also known as erethism, was first considered to be a psychosis particularly common to hat makers, becoming known as "mad hatter's disease." For centuries, mercury was used in the treatment of furs used for hat making. The presumed-to-be psychological symptoms included mental confusion, emotional disturbance, poor memory, shyness, nervousness, insomnia, tremors, lack of coordination, and dizziness. However, with removal of mercury from the physical body, psychological disturbance disappears. The disease was then, and is now, a treatable medical condition affecting neurology and thus behavior.[24]

Fibromyalgia and chronic fatigue syndrome are often referred to as diseases with "unknown etiology," suggesting a psychological rather than physical origin of symptoms. But this unknown is only and precisely a lack of knowledge of the physical causes of disease.

The psychiatrist Thomas Szasz has compared the diagnosis of physical illness as mental illness as similar to condemnation during the fifteenth century witch trials. No actual proof is required, and the diagnostician often makes up justifications

---

[22] See: *Clinical Medicine and Research*, Kumar et al., found at
http://www.ncbi.nlm.nih.gov/pmc/articles/PMC3064755/

[23] *Epilepsia*, Vol. 44, Suppl. 6, 2003.

[24] Found at http://en.wikipedia.org/wiki/Mad_hatter_disease.

based on ignorance or financial gain. Szasz observed that a main complaint against psychiatric diagnosis and involuntary mental hospitalization is "that patients are committed too often and too readily—for example, that patients with unrecognized bodily diseases . . . are sometimes hastily categorized as (neurotic or) psychotic and improperly confined."[25]

When people are seriously ill and treated as if they are not, the experience is *shaming*. Richard Kradin, a physician who believes illnesses such as fibromyalgia and chronic fatigue syndrome are psychosomatic makes this observation: "There is no group of patients in medical practice as disparaged as those with psychosomatic disorders. They are pejoratively labeled by doctors as 'crocks,' shunned, and at times even psychologically sadistically abused by otherwise well-intentioned caregivers."[26] Kradin emphasizes that patients and their families must be told that the pain and suffering are simply illusion, and that medical testing to discover underlying physical causes should be discouraged. What he proposes amounts to misleading patients when he says: "The best pragmatic compromise is to begin by simply acknowledging that a patient's symptoms are 'real' but unexplained, leaving their ultimate cause for future discussion."[27] This "further discussion" is intended to convince the patients that their illness is not real.

Few situations are more shaming than being tricked and misled by the very professionals we have entrusted with our health and well-being. The denial of testing to determine actual causes of illness only prolongs suffering, delaying measures that could potentially improve patient quality of life. This approach to the ill essentially disempowers patients and

[25] Thomas Szasz, *The Manufacture of Madness: A Comparative Study of the Inquisition and the Mental Health Movement*, Harper and Row, New York, 1970, p. 25.
[26] Kradin, Richard, *Pathologies of the Mind/Body Interface: Exploring the Curious Domain of the Psychosomatic Disorders,* Routledge, New York, 2013, pp. 128-129.
[27] *Ibid.*, p. 123.

fosters a relationship of dominance that hinders healing. Dishonesty toward patients is tantamount to disrespecting and shaming them.

Medical ignorance of the presence of physical disease is not proof of mental illness. It is a result of a lack of information and understanding. Serious ethical questions are raised when the physical suffering of patients is ignored or translated into presumed psychiatric disorder. For example, family practitioner Patrick Wood, MD, explains in a YouTube lecture that he initially wanted to prove that fibromyalgia patients were psychiatrically ill. However, the more he learned about the real pain of the disease, the more his opinion changed. He initiated significant research that fosters treating patients with respect and explores medical solutions to alleviate their suffering. Now he counsels patients this way: "If a clinician says 'I don't believe in fibromyalgia, it doesn't exist,' you have my permission to laugh in their face, and by all means, get yourself a different doctor!"[28]

Finding respectful, informed health care practitioners is essential for patients in pain. This can be a daunting endeavor, especially during times of diminished energy and capacity. Health care professionals can be authoritarian in their approach to patients, a style that may or may not suit individual needs. Becoming informed about your condition is crucial. At times you may be placed in the difficult position of determining whether a recommended medication or treatment might actually be beneficial. And side effects must always be weighed. Many people in pain report that their doctors are unable or unwilling to take the time to learn about their particular condition and concerns. I often hear patients in

---

[28] *Wood, Patrick M.D., Fibromyalgia: New Insights, New Hope,* https://www.youtubebe.com/watch?v=XLvcA6Xhzas. *This is Part Three of the series. Part one is at https://youtube.com/watch?v=iL4pMWa351M and Part Two is at https:www.youtube/watch?v=Fc1dw/TLQ0F4.*

pain complain that they have had to become their own doctors. They know more about their condition than their trained professionals who either have not been properly educated or have failed to keep up to date as new knowledge becomes available. It may be helpful to bring significant articles to your doctors so that they may learn about the information that is important to you. If this gesture meets resistance or resentment, perhaps it is time to find someone more amenable to your needs.

Research in the last thirty years has opened new doors to knowledge regarding severe chronic pain. Brain scans and other tests have revealed a mechanism quite different from the familiar one that registers traumatic pain from, for example, a broken bone or a burn. In the case of "central sensitization," the central nervous system becomes activated to produce pain and remains in that state. Biochemical changes in cells, the brain, and spinal fluid keep pain levels abnormally high. This type of pain is body-wide and without apparent external cause. As a result of this breakthrough, new research has focused on bringing the brain and central nervous system back to normal levels, thereby quelling the pain. Drugs such as low-dose naltrexone and others are proving successful in giving sufferers of chronic pain a better quality of life. The future becomes brighter for us all.

My personal journey with pain is still challenging but there have been significant improvements. I have been fortunate to find doctors willing to listen and to try new treatments. I have learned that exercise is an indispensible part of pain management. Bodies need to move and stretch to stay healthy. Even when pain is severe, simply moving your hands, feet, arms and legs rhythmically while lying in bed or sitting in a chair can increase levels of natural endorphins and reduce pain. When possible, I prefer to walk or jog for exercise, but if pain interferes, playing favorite music and dancing while sitting is fun and energizing.

Laughter, learning, and friends are great distractions from pain. They may not cure illness, but they make difficult times a good deal more tolerable. Perhaps most important for healing is maintaining the hope that progress will continue and the future will offer the cures that elude us today.

* * *

Bonnie Scot: Bachelor of Science, Biology; M.A., Depth Psychology; Ph.D. Candidate, Depth Psychology; Facilitator, Santa Barbara Sansum Clinic Fibromyalgia and Chronic Fatigue Syndrome Information and Support Group.

At this point, I will offer my own personal perspective on psychosomatic illness in the hope that what I have to say will ring a resonant bell in you. At best, it may seem self-evident. At least, it may cause you to reexamine your beliefs.

By way of preface, I want to report an intriguing, totally unexpected and recent phenomenon that has an uncanny connection to this topic:

> *I have just had a flare-up of fibromyalgia! This is happening after three or four years of this condition being under the radar – meaning manageable and unproblematic. Many of the physical symptoms I described earlier in Part One[29] I began to reexperience during the time I was writing Part One. The soreness in my feet made it hard to walk and the pain in my fingers made it hard to type. My neck and shoulders were hurting again. I was asking myself: "Why is this happening? Why is it happening now?" Certainly, there*

---

[29] Cf. above, pp. 8 - 10.

were some possible external causes to be considered including my long hospitalization and surgery, the big drop in temperature in the evenings, and the rain. Any or all of these may have played a part. But what stood out starkly staring me in the face was the fact that I was thinking about, writing about, and focusing on pain. And voila! There it was. A clear case of psychosomatic illness.

I stopped writing to see if that would make a difference. It did not. It could be that I didn't stop for long enough. Even more to the point, however, was the obvious fact that whether or not I was writing, I was still thinking about it. Was my thinking about pain enough to cause it? If it was still on my mind, was it my mind that was making me ill? And if that was so, does it mean that I was right - quite literally - when, as explained in the preface, I had put off writing this book on the basis that a book on pain is painful. When the book is finished, it will be interesting to see whether the pain will be finished too.

Although I cannot delve into the complexities of the theoretical debate on this issue, I will focus on a few essential points that, hopefully, will be sufficient for our purposes. After the dust of disputation has cleared, these are the key elements we need to keep in mind. I will share what I *know* to be true and what I *believe* to be true about psychosomatic illness.

First, what I know is that *the pain is real*. It is not in my head; it is in my body. It is not feigned or intentionally produced (as in Malingering or Factitious Disorder.) And I believe this will most likely hold true for the estimated *five million* people in the United States who suffer with this condition.

Second, it is *not under any conscious control*. It is not chosen and it cannot be stopped by an act of will. Therefore, it makes no sense to hold patients responsible or blame them for their condition. Treating them as if they can do what they are clearly unable to do – such as trying to force them to eat or walk or climb stairs – is not only futile; it is destructive to the patient. It cannot be condoned.

Third, people who are sick and in pain deserve medical treatment, regardless of whether there are psychological factors that affect the onset or duration of their condition. Although the organic causes may not be known in the present, this does not rule out the possibility that they will be discovered in the future. Such is the history of medical science.

At one time, it was believed that illnesses were caused by evil spirits or by visitations by the devil or by punishments by God for wrong-doing. We consider it "progress" that we can now identify organic causes for the majority of illnesses. Hence, it is reasonable to suppose that as our science progresses, new information about the causes, viable treatments and even cures may be revealed for those illnesses currently regarded as "psychosomatic." Perhaps this term should be understood to indicate more about the boundaries of our current medical knowledge than as a denigration of those unfortunates suffering with illnesses.

Consider the following portrait of a patient with a psychosomatic illness. The author, a practicing pulmonologist and psychoanalyst at Massachusetts General Hospital, has this to say:

"The severity of symptoms in the absence of objective abnormalities, her reported side effects in response to multiple drugs, her irritable affect, and the intensity of her negative reaction to being told that she was not suffering from an organic disease, are all ... characteristic of psychosomatic patients. Yet her upset is readily understood as patients with psychosomatic disorders, by definition, locate their discomfort in their bodies, not in their minds, and resist the notion that their perceptions might be incorrect."[30]

With this unflattering picture, it is difficult to imagine that a physician looking through such a narrowed lens would be capable of respect and compassion for these patients. He is convinced of his absolute rightness and, borrowing his own words, he "resists the notion that [his] perceptions might be incorrect." It is exactly this attitude of disrespect and arrogance that is the source of patients' complaints.

It is understandably frustrating for physicians to be unable to help their patients. They *want* to be successful. And it is human, albeit unacceptable, to avoid their own feelings of failure by projecting them on the patient rather than accepting the limitations of their own knowledge. Nonetheless, blaming the patient only makes a bad situation worse.

Further, I believe it is not coincidental but highly significant that most of the patients diagnosed with psychosomatic illnesses are *women*. For example, of the United States population, 3.5% of women and .516% of males are believed to have fibromyalgia. The treating physicians, on the other hand, are overwhelmingly male. I believe what we are seeing here is a political issue: it is rooted in sexist discrimination against women.

Stereotypically, women are regarded as overly emotional, hysterical,[31] and prone to be victims. They are frequently treated with frustration and contempt based on these qualities. However, we can entertain a very different interpretation of these so-called typical female qualities. It might be that women are more tuned into their emotions, more

---

[30] Kradin, Richard L., *Pathologies of the Mind/Body Interface: Exploring the Curious Domain of the Psychosomatic Disorders,* Routledge, New York, 2013, Introduction, p. xvi.

[31] Freud regarded as "hysterical" many of his female patients who reported sexual abuse. Perhaps they were speaking the truth and it was Freud who was unable to accept the prevalence of sexual abuse in his day.

sensitive to their bodies, and more integrated in their mind/body connection. What has been traditionally regarded as a deficit can be reframed as an advantage. It all depends on who is making the evaluation.

My final point, stated somewhat provocatively, is: *All illness is psychosomatic.* The term "psychosomatic" unites psyche and soma in one word just as human beings unite psyche and soma in one person. It is impossible to separate mind and body in Cartesian fashion. Human beings are organic wholes.

We all know, for instance, that worry can cause headaches and pain in our bodies can alter our mood. Mind and body interact constantly. Earlier[32] we saw that, according to the ACE study, abuse and neglect in childhood can create a predisposition for organic disease in adulthood. Trauma gets locked in the nervous system and can be reactivated in situations that occur years later. Thus, in EMDR therapy,[33] we need to work with beliefs, feelings AND bodily symptoms to release trauma and allow people to heal.

In his latest book, Bessel Van der Kolk states:

"While we all want to move beyond trauma, the part of our brain that is devoted to ensuring our survival (deep below our rational brain) is not very good at denial. Long after a traumatic experience is over, it may be reactivated at the slightest hint of danger and mobilize disturbed brain circuits and secrete massive amounts of stress hormones. This precipitates unpleasant emotions, intense physical sensations, and impulsive and aggressive actions. These post traumatic reactions feel incomprehensible and overwhelming. Feeling out of control, survivors of trauma often begin to fear that they are damaged to the core and beyond redemption."[34]

---

[32] Cf. above, p. 12.

[33] See my previous book, *Therapy at Lightning Speed: Case Studies of EMDR,* Journey Press, Santa Barbara, 2011.

[34] Van Der Kolk, M.D., Bessel:, *The Body Keeps the Score: Brain, Mind, and Body in the Healing of Trauma,* Viking press, New York, 2014, p. 2.

Then Dr. Van der Kolk adds: "We now know that their behaviors are not the result of moral failings or signs of lack of willpower or bad character – they are caused by actual changes in the brain."[35]

In the end, it is only by acknowledging and treating *all* aspects of a human being – the physical, emotional, mental, behavioral, and spiritual – that we can hope to heal those in pain.

* * *

---

[35] *Ibid.*, p. 3.

PART THREE:

Rising Above

Working with Pain

We have visited in depth the essential components of the pain experience and how it simultaneously affects both the body and the mind in a myriad of negative ways. Now it is time to address the compelling question: What are we to do about it? How can sufferers learn to live with their pain in the most constructive and promising manner? How can caregivers guide their patients toward acceptance and, whenever possible, the reduction and relief of pain?

1. Being on your own side

While it is natural to turn against the body when it causes us to suffer such intense agony, it is not helpful to do so. It is like waving a cape at a raging bull: it just causes it to charge even more fiercely. It is incumbent on us to learn to quiet the raging bull and, as Tara Brach says: "to move from fight/flight to tend and befriend."[36]

According to Brach, illness may be understood as being down on oneself and identifying with a sense of deficiency – the belief that "something is wrong with me" – rather than supporting oneself with a compassionate attitude expressed in her words: "It's okay, sweetheart."[37]

One way is through mindfulness meditation where we simply notice what is happening in the moment and allow it to be. We pay attention to the physical sensations of pain while

[36] Brach, Tara: *Deliberate Practice and Inner Transformation,* Psychotherapy Networker webinar, December 2014.
[37] *Ibid.*

practising an attitude of openness, kindness and non-judgment. In this process, we move toward a more peaceful coexistence with what is hurting and transform resistance into acceptance of the experience of pain. This is currently a very popular approach.

I myself use a different approach to shift from self-attack to self-love and compassion. It involves learning to silence the critical voice inside which I call the "superego,"[38] that part inside that is not your friend.

We all have a voice inside which criticizes and condemns, attacks and berates us. It represents the internalization of negative messages we received about ourselves originating in our families of origin and carried forward in time through our own thought processes. This voice was there in the background when, in Part One, we spoke about feeling guilty for the irritation and grumpiness which often accompanies illness and the constant presence of pain.[39] It was present behind the scenes in the description of the shame of being seen as a person in pain, someone different from and less than healthy people.[40] And it has been there in my mind since I wrote about the recent flare-up of fibromyalgia I experienced during the writing of Part One.[41] The possibility of its being "psychosomatic" conjured up a superego image of myself as neurotic, histrionic or, in some undefined way, psychologically damaged. It made me feel bad about myself.

Then, when I trouped off to Italy still in the throes of a fibro flare-up, I began to doubt myself. Was I an intrepid warrior who refused to give up or a pathetic cripple limping my way down cobble-stoned streets revealing my helplessness

---

[38] See Aarons, Rachel: *Journey to Home: Quintessential Therapy and Beyond*, Part 3, Silencing the Superego, pp. 69 - 100, Journey Press, Santa Barbara, 2009.

[39] See above, Part One, p. 12.

[40] See above, Part One, p. 14.

[41] See above, Part Two, p. 120.

to the world? The superego took the latter, considerably less appealing point of view.

What I practice myself and what I teach my clients is not to succumb to the superego but to fight back. Ways to do this vary from undermining the authority of the superego, recognizing the manipulative ploy of the superego, identifying the source of this strategy in our family of origin, denying the truth of the message we are receiving, or bypassing the message entirely by affirming the self. With each client, we identify the specific superego messages they are receiving on a regular basis and then we go through a series of proposed counter-attacks until we find the ones that are the most effective for each specific individual. The way you will know that a particular counter–attack is effective is the fact that, at least temporarily, the superego voice goes silent. Then, for a brief time, the mind is empty.

In this spaciousness, we cultivate a new and different voice that advocates for the self. I call it the "sympathetic witness." It is an inner voice that is on your side, holding your best interests, and treating you with loving kindness. It is, no doubt, the voice that Tara Brach quotes as saying to herself: "It's okay, sweetheart."

The implication is that, as well as the various outside people who provide care to the patient, there needs to be a caregiver *inside* each person in pain, who is the kind of empathic caregiver we were promoting in Part Two. From this perspective, Part One and Part Two may be regarded as addressing the same person.

The more you hear this compassionate voice in place of the critical superego voice, the more centered and peaceful you will feel. Being on your own side is an essential step to integrating a self divided.

I think Tom's story speaks meaningfully on this point.

Compassionate Caregiving From a Distance: Tom Robinson

Because I am a life coach for people who are living with chronic illnesses and chronic pain, and am in a relationship with a woman who for the last 18 months has been living with severe chronic pain from osteoarthritis, rheumatoid arthritis, osteoporosis, fibromyalgia, and restless leg syndrome, I thought it would be relatively easy for me to write a chapter for this book.

I was wrong. Before I explain why, and before I tell you how Mary Ellen's illnesses and chronic pain have made our relationship much more difficult and challenging, I want to give you some background information to provide a context for this chapter.

I help Mary Ellen as much as I am able. But because I work full time and because we are in a long distance relationship (we live about 60 miles apart), I am not able to be her caretaker. But I think there are many aspects of our story that caregivers and people living with chronic pain will find both interesting and helpful.

Our relationship is somewhat unusual. Because of our childhood wounds and other reasons, it has been very difficult. In the five years since we met, we have gone through several break-ups. But love, and a sense that we are meant to be together, brought us back together after each one. Over the past five years, we have both learned a lot and grown a lot, and we're both working hard to have a relationship that works.

Getting back to the reasons I was wrong when I thought it would be relatively easy to write this chapter, the biggest one is something that Rachel wrote about in the Reflections On Pain section. The process of writing it has made it impossible for me to deny the possibility that the time may come when

Mary Ellen decides her pain is so great and her quality of life is so poor, that she does not want to continue living.

I hope that time never comes. I hope she finds a combination of treatments that lessen her pain enough that she can get an adequate amount of sleep and not continue to suffer. As someone who, because of working with hundreds of people with chronic illnesses and because of living and dealing with a chronic illness myself (Crohn's disease), is knowledgeable about both alternative and standard medicine, I know there are many treatments Mary Ellen can try.

But none of the treatments, diet changes, supplements, etc. she has tried so far has brought about a significant improvement. So the possibility that at some point she will stop trying to get better and decide she does not want to continue living appears to me to be a very real one.

While I have been able to stay in denial about the possibility of Mary Ellen wanting to end her life, I have been very aware of another challenge of being in a relationship with her. That challenge, and it's a hard one, is the helplessness I feel when I know that she is in a lot of pain, while I also know there is nothing I can do to lessen it.

I want to say here that I believe in and have come to know a God that loves each one of us more than we can possibly imagine. But when I see someone suffering and in frequent and oftentimes constant pain, especially someone whom I love and who is a very important person in my life, I can't help but wonder why God would allow that to happen. Maybe someday I will learn the answer, but I know it's possible that I never will.

I have learned firsthand that it is much easier to coach someone who is living with chronic illness and pain than it is to be in an intimate relationship with someone who is. But there is one thing Mary Ellen does that goes a long way in counter-balancing the difficult feelings I experience that I have shared with you. And it's a very simple thing: she tells me how much she appreciates the things I do for her.

Whether those things are big or small, when she notices them and lets me know how much of a difference they make in her life, I feel good inside. Her appreciation doesn't make all the angst I have from the difficult challenges I've described go away, but it goes a long way in mitigating it and deepening our connection.

One other thing Mary Ellen does that helps me a lot is to ask me how I'm doing and how my day is going. She doesn't always do that, and given how much pain she is often in, I can understand why she would sometimes forget. But I sure appreciate it when she remembers.

Now that I've told you about the hardest challenges I deal with because of Mary Ellen's chronic illness and pain, I want to switch gears and tell you about a very effective way to lessen the emotional pain that comes with virtually all difficult challenges in life, including having a chronic illness or chronic pain, and also caring for someone who does.

One of this way's biggest advantages is that it does not depend on anyone else. You can do it for yourself virtually anytime and anywhere.

What I am referring to is self-compassion.

You may be wondering why I'm saying that self-compassion is so helpful, or how to give it to yourself, or both. If so, here are the answers to those questions.

One of the easiest ways to give yourself self-compassion is the following: Imagine that someone you care about deeply is living with the same challenge or pain that you are. That person can be a close friend, a partner, a spouse, a parent, or someone else. Or, if you're a parent, you can imagine that your child has grown up, and is living and trying to deal with and manage a situation like yours.

When you picture the person you care about facing the same angst you do, and experiencing the same pain—physical or emotional or both—that you are, you will, as I have learned from leading hundreds of people through this exercise, be deeply touched, and you will have strong feelings of compassion and empathy for them.

The next step is to go into the bathroom with those feelings of empathy and compassion, and look into the mirror. As you do, look into that person's eyes. You will see the pain (again, physical or emotional or both) that they are in and you will see that they deserve lots and lots of compassion.

Send it to that person in the mirror, from your heart and through your soft eyes. And if it feels right, you can talk to them too. Finally, feel the peace and healing inside yourself from the compassion you've just received.

We all need compassion when we are in any kind of significant pain, but a lot of the time we don't get it. Not only that, but when painful things happen to us, many of us make the pain we feel even worse by blaming ourselves for it. But now you know a much better response. I hope you will use it often.

*   *   *

Tom Robinson, M.A., is a life coach who works with people who are struggling or overwhelmed by chronic illness. You can find out more about him or get his free e-course via his website: www.chronicillnesscoach.com.

2. Focusing on the positive

We have seen that the more you focus on pain, the more pain you feel. Sometimes we may have no choice when pain takes over every fiber of our being. But when it is possible, it is helpful to put our focus elsewhere.

During the long ordeal in hospital, I often needed a way to raise my spirits and find something positive to focus on. My son and I frequently downloaded movies to watch on our computer. We brought in dinner from outside and ate it out on the patio with a vase of flowers on the table. We found a cache of chocolate bars tucked away in a drawer on one of the wards and turned that into a treat to look forward to. But the best time by far happened on a night that was particularly grueling for me. On the edge of despair, I complained to my son that I really needed something to lift me up. It was feeling all too much for me. He found a desk chair on wheels, plunked me down on it, and pushed me up and down a deserted corridor at break neck speed, wheeling me around as I howled with laughter. That was an amazing feat of ingenuity on his part.

When it is a matter of focus, hypnosis is a powerful tool for teaching us to focus our attention where we want it to be and not where the mind tends to take it. Also known as "selective perception," hypnosis allows us to go to our own special place that is tranquil and calming where we can deeply relax.[42] To the extent that we are able to relax, we will feel less pain.

In contrast to many practitioners who teach self-hypnosis, I train my clients in deepening techniques in addition to basic methodology so they can choose the level of hypnotic state that is needed in the moment. Basic methodology will work for average circumstances but, for the aversive ones, we may need to go deeper in order, as in the case in point, to get beyond severe pain.

In addition, there are pain reduction methods that utilize self-hypnosis to regulate the desired level of our pain. Here are

---

[42] My hypnosis process is available on my website as an audio download if you scroll down on the page "What is Hypnosis?" or in tape and CD form through my office [See Contact Information at the end of the book.]

some examples. We can visualize being below the level of our pain by imagining ourselves warm and dry in a burrow at the bottom of a river while the pain churns above us like a raging river. Or, we can float above it like a cloud in the sky while our body lies on the bed below. Or, as another alternative, we can put the pain at a distance from us by projecting it on to a TV screen while we operate the remote control. We can pause it or fast forward it or turn it off altogether.

Another favorite technique is "color bath" in which we imagine bringing a soothing color down from the top of our heads into each muscle and organ of our body. If any area resists, we let the color play around and in and out of the area of tension as if we were massaging ourselves with soothing, healing color.

Finally, a very effective technique is to begin by identifying the qualities of the pain we are experiencing – the size, shape, texture, temperature, and associated imagery – and then proceed to change these qualities to ones that are more benign and comfortable. For example, a back pain that is six inches across, shaped like a picket fence with sharp edges and a rough surface, that is boring into our muscles like iron spikes may be converted into one that is, say, two inches across, soft, smooth, and more like a warm hand on our back. As an interesting note, most people choose to keep a small amount of pain and not eliminate it entirely, perhaps to remind themselves to be careful or, perhaps, because they have become identified with the pain and can't imagine completely letting it go.

In this regard, author Rick Hanson explains how the brain is predisposed to negativity and will retain negative experiences in long term memory while positive experiences wash through and are forgotten.[43] This "negativity bias," as he terms it, is rooted in our biological need for survival. The amygdala is

---

[43] Hanson, Rick: *Buddha's Brain: The Practical Neuroscience of Happiness, Love & Wisdom,* New Harbinger Publications, Oakland, California, 2009, p. 68.

constantly scanning for threats of harm to the organism and keeps this information in implicit memory to arm and protect us. In his words, the negative experiences are like "Velcro" to the brain whereas positive experiences are like "Teflon." However, according to Hanson, we can learn to reverse this tendency and turn passing mental states into stable neural traits in order to benefit ourselves and other beings.[44] He offers recommendations for locking in positive experiences so that they become a solid part of who we are and inform our sense of self through memory. As psychologist Donald Hebb is often quoted as saying: "Neurons that fire together wire together."[45] In other words, it is what we focus on that becomes real for us. Hence it is important, in Hanson's words, to "take in the good" – that is, to ensure that the positive experiences of each day are committed to memory. As the title of his latest book suggests,[46] we are, in effect, "hardwiring happiness." As a result, we will experience more self-esteem and less depression, more pleasure and less pain.

Hanson says: "Given the negativity bias of the brain, it takes an *active* effort to internalize positive experiences and heal negative ones. When you tilt toward what is positive, you're actually righting a neurological imbalance. And you're giving yourself today the caring and encouragement you should have received as a child, but perhaps didn't receive in full measure."[47]

If we recall the results of the ACE study that we talked about in Part One[48] about how adverse experiences in childhood lead to mental and physical illnesses in adulthood,

[44] Hanson, Rick: *Brain Science and Psychotherapy: What's the Next Step?*, Psychotherapy Networker Symposium, Keynote Address, 2014.

[45] Quoted in Hanson, Rick: *Buddha's Brain*, p. 68.

[46] Hanson, Rick Ph.D, *Hardwiring Happiness: The New Brain Science of Contentment, Calm and Confidence*, Harmony Books, New York, 2013.

[47] *Ibid.*, p. 75.

[48] See above, p. 12.

this approach can be seen as offsetting the effects of early childhood abuse and neglect by installing new positive feelings that become part of the structure of the brain. "Consequently, positive feelings have far-reaching benefits including a stronger immune system and a cardiovascular system that is less reactive to stress. They lift your mood; increase optimism, resilience and resourcefulness; and help counteract the effects of painful experiences, including trauma."[49] Focusing on the positive shifts the balance away from pain and illness in the direction of health and well-being.

3. What is your passion?

Many of us have interests, hobbies and activities that are passions for us. They absorb our attention and keep us wholly captivated, sometimes for hours at a time. As we engage in our special passion, we may lose track of time entirely. And what is most important, we may lose awareness of our bodily pain, either wholly or in part.

This passion could be an art form such as painting, sculpture, or ceramics. It could be a physical activity such as boating, golf or gardening. For myself, when I am able to garden, I get totally immersed in the earth. I love seeing the changes appear before my eyes as the weeds disappear and the flowers are planted. Hours fly by before my body reminds me that enough is enough – or it *was* an hour or more ago.

I am also reminded of a woman I know whose body has been in constant pain for many years. While she could barely move without suffering, she lost all perception of pain when she got up and danced with her seniors' singing and dancing group. Seeing her up on stage performing the intricate and

---

[49] Hanson, Rick: p.75 citing Frederickson (2000), Frederickson and Levenson (1998), Frederickson (2001), Frederickson et al. (2000).

demanding moves of the dance routine, you would never suspect that she suffered severe chronic pain.

Like dancing, music is known to transport people into an altered state, whether they are listening or performing. Similarly, many people lose themselves in reading. In books, they are living in other worlds beyond their own. All these passions give us a reprieve, a window of time in which pain disappears, or at least recedes, from the center of our awareness.

This reprieve can also come from putting our focus on others. Sometimes we just need to get out of ourselves for a while. When I am doing therapy, for example, I forget my own pain as I become present and engaged with my clients. In the same way, volunteer work is a great way to make a shift from self-absorption to connection with others. To volunteer your services is a way to provide benefit to another and escape from yourself at the same time.

The same shift often happens when we are spending time with friends or family, participating fully in the conversation or enjoying a shared activity. Laughter detaches us and elevates us in the same movement. Having fun with people who matter to us offers a much-needed and welcome release from pain.

According to Bessel Van der Kolk:

"Being able to feel safe with other people is the single most important aspect of mental health… Numerous studies of disaster responses around the globe have shown that social support is the most powerful protection against becoming overwhelmed by stress and trauma."[50]

However, he goes on to clarify:

"Social support is not the same as merely being in the presence of others. The critical issue is *reciprocity:* being truly

---

[50] Van der Kolk, Bessel M.D., *The Body Keeps the Score*, p. 79.

heard and seen by the people around us, feeling that we are held in someone's mind and heart. For our physiology to calm down, heal, and grow, we need a visceral feeling of safety. No doctor can write a prescription for friendship and love."[51]

It is not surprising, then, that people with strong social networks that offer them support of this kind are more likely to heal and heal faster than those with the same illnesses who are socially isolated and alone.

This experience of support from an attuned other can come from friends and family. It can also come, as we have seen, from the caregivers that are looking after us. Some doctors and nurses are intuitively aware of how to help their patients feel seen and heard. This can make all the difference for us. When people around us, either personal or professional, are able to offer this sense of presence and safety, when their gestures of help really *are* helpful, it is important to let them know. They deserve our encouragement and appreciation. We need to be as responsive to them as we want them to be to us. Support is a two-way street.

Lastly, millions of people around the world find relief and comfort in their religious beliefs and spiritual practices. Being connected to a church, temple or mosque provides a link to others in the congregation – a community of like minds – while it also connects us to the divine. Daily practices of prayer and meditation offer ways to remind us that there is a transcendent reality and broader purpose beyond our ordinary limited perspective. Feeling that there is a higher power who cares about our suffering may imbue us with the strength to tolerate adversity and the comfort of a benevolent spirit who is always there to turn to. An abiding experience of God or godliness can take us through the dark night of the soul and help us rise above our pain.

---

[51] *Ibid.*.

4. Releasing the negative

As a counterpoint to increasing the positive experiences that come to form a part of our sense of self, we can also work on releasing the negative experiences that have been interfering with our ability to live a happy and productive life. Prime examples are traumatic experiences - that is to say, experiences that were overwhelming to the individual in terms of the structures they had available at the time. Such experiences may not hit the headlines of the newspaper as do earthquakes, floods and other natural disasters, horrors of war, or human atrocities. They may be everyday events in our lives that become locked in the nervous system and limbic area of the brain, events that seem stuck in time and cannot be processed through. When circumstances arise that trigger these unprocessed memories, we find ourselves responding as if the original trauma in the past were happening again in the present.

As Bessel van der Kolk points out: "One does not have to be a combat soldier or visit a refugee camp in Syria or the Congo to encounter trauma. Trauma happens to us, our friends, our families, and our neighbors. Research by the Centers for Disease Control and Prevention has shown that one in five Americans was sexually molested as a child; one in four was beaten by a parent to the point of a mark being left on their body; and one in three couples engages in physical violence. A quarter of us grew up with alcoholic relatives, and one out of eight witnessed their mother being beaten or hit."[52] Trauma is all around us.

In my professional opinion, by far the fastest and most effective way of releasing trauma and reprocessing unresolved memories is EMDR therapy. The description of EMDR in the

---

[52] Van Der Kolk M.D., Bessel: *The Body Keeps the Score*, p. 1.

World Health Organization's recent guidelines for treating stress condition reads as follows:

"Eye movement desensitization and reprocessing (EMDR): This therapy is based on the idea that negative thoughts, feelings, and behaviors are the result of unprocessed memories. The treatment involves standardized procedures that include focusing simultaneously on (a)spontaneous associations of traumatic images, thoughts, emotions, and bodily sensations and (b)bilateral stimulation that is most commonly in the form of repeated eye movements.[53]

I have been so impressed with the speed and efficacy of EMDR therapy that I wrote a book about it.[54] In this book, you will see a series of case studies of EMDR therapy that I have done addressing a variety of different problems including acute recent trauma, major depression, rage attacks, self-sabotage in business, submissiveness, despair, couples' interlocking pathologies, and social anxiety. Since that time, I have done EMDR therapy with a multitude of other problems and it has consistently facilitated breakthroughs in each and every case. It has been nothing short of remarkable.

I will share a few words about a case in point that is immediately relevant to the concerns of this book.

Several years ago, I saw a woman with a staggering number of diverse somatic and psychic symptoms stemming, she believed, from early childhood abuse. Her symptom list included:

- high blood pressure,
- incontinence,
- endometriosis,
- rosacea,

---

[53] Quoted in: EMDRIA Newsletter: The Information Resource for EMDR Therapists, Vol. 19, Issue 4, December 2014, p. 5.

[54] Aarons, Rachel B., *Therapy at Lightning Speed: Case Studies of EMDR*, Journey Press, Santa Barbara California, 2011.

- tinnitus,
- nerve pain in her feet,
- melanoma in her shoulder,
- basal cell carcinoma on her nose,
- squamous cell carcinoma in her leg,
- problem with tear ducts & mid-range depth perception in her eyes,
- two surgeries for lateral imbalance in her eyes,
- shattered teeth from grinding her teeth at night,
- losing balance & breaking bones,
- difficulty swallowing,
- back problems,
- a series of plastic surgeries because she hated her body,
- panic attacks where she couldn't move or breathe,
- anxiety with city noise & movement,
- mood swings,
- lack of boundaries,
- persistent feeling of emptiness,
- clinical depression.

You have to admit this is an extraordinarily long list that constitutes a devastating history of both physical and mental pain and suffering.

Traumatic memories of her child abuse had been accessed through hypnotherapy and prior psychotherapy going back more than thirty years. As a foundational event, she recalled her mother attempting to smother her as an infant in her crib to stop her from crying. When her father came in to save her, her mother said: "I hate her!" She had carried this feeling of being despised and unwanted her entire life.

Her first EMDR therapy was geared toward her stated goal of "relieving the feeling of terror and unsafety I feel when confronted with sound, vibration, and a shadow of something bigger than me." The negative belief she had internalized was: "It's my fault if my life is in danger." She had learned as an infant that she had to be quiet and good to survive because her mother did not want to feed her or change her very often. Hence, being aware of her needs and being assertive about them was a lifelong problem for her. The conclusion she had drawn and lived out through her childhood and adulthood was that, if she was unwanted, she must have deserved it. Her symptom list was a testimony to her self-hate.

In the processing, she was able to enact a confrontation with her mother about her dismally poor parenting skills and come to the recognition that the responsibility lay with her mother, not with herself. In place of the harsh introduction to the world she had had in reality, she was able, in imagination, to have a corrective experience of being born in what she called "a cocoon of love" with two nurturing and supportive figures in her life. The experience, she reported, was "ecstatic" for her. She had never had the feeling of being wanted before. "It was a total reset," she said.

This was not the only trauma in this woman's life, nor was it the end of her therapy. There were scars on her back that her mother said had come from diaper pins but which the doctor said were cigarette burns. She was sexually abused by her alcoholic father while her mother watched. They were, in her words, "partners in crime." When she had pain with urination, her mother examined her invasively to look for tears in the tissues and then refused to take her to a doctor, insisting there were no tears. She felt used as a "prop" for her mother's image in the world and became perfectionistic in her demands on herself. Despite becoming a successful CEO of her company, nothing she did seemed good enough.

As we continued to work, symptoms began to reveal their messages about the wants and needs she was not expressing in her life. For example, a bout of incontinence she experienced when friends from out of town stayed an uncomfortably long time came to an end the day they left. Similarly, once she associated the noise and vibration with the nickel factory located beside her house when she was an infant, she was able to tolerate being in big cities. Gradually, the symptoms receded. As trauma was addressed and released, they were not needed anymore.

As in apparent in this example, EMDR therapy is not just about releasing negative experiences. It also provides opportunities for positive advances. As trauma becomes desensitized, new options appear in the reprocessing of memories. The client opens to seeing new ways of being they were blocked from seeing before. The work known as "future template" allows them to visualize in detail the ways they will handle things in the future very differently than they did in the past. It exemplifies the changes in feelings, thoughts and behavior that were goals of the work. It moves the client from the self that was stuck in trauma to the person they want and need to be.

A case I worked on very recently is illuminating in regard to demonstrating how pain can operate as a block to forward movement. The young woman in question experienced a traumatic accident on an airplane when a suitcase fell down from an upper bin and landed right on top of her. She woke up in shock and excruciating pain. The airline crew were decidedly unsympathetic and unhelpful. Since that unfortunate event, she has had years of medical procedures with minimal improvement. She remains stuck in extreme pain.

The timing of this accident was particularly unfortunate for her. It happened at a peak time of her life. She had just completed her bar examination to become an attorney, had a successful business, and was planning to get married. She felt that the world was her oyster and she was capable of achieving anything she wanted. All this drastically changed on that airplane.

She has not been able to practice law, continue her business, or get married. Her life was stopped in its tracks just at the point when everything was working perfectly for her.

Now it seemed to her as if all roads were blocked. Further, she comes from a culture where independence is highly revered. The last thing she could tolerate was being "a victim." This idea was abhorrent to her. Hence she suppressed her feelings and kept her sadness and anger inside. She soldiered on, never complaining or admitting just how badly she felt. In her mind, all she wished for was to get back the life she had lost.

During the processing, it became evident that any time we tried to get to the feeling level, some part of her body would react with a high level of pain. Then the pain would command her full attention and the feelings would be pushed aside. We had to counter this bodily blockade.

Using her imagination and the power of the unconscious mind, she was able, repeatedly, to relieve the pain in each area of her body as it came up. We were then free to address the feelings that lay beneath it. What became apparent was that the pain was acting as a defense to prevent her from moving forward in her life. She was consumed with looking back in time. Admittedly, her life would not be exactly as she had envisioned it and, undoubtedly, it would take time for her to recreate a semblance of what it had been. But we came to the realization that, with "baby steps" she could make her life meaningful. There was hope for a positive future for her if she was willing to accept it.

5. Embracing Love

We have looked at releasing negative experiences that were intimately entwined with our pain experience. This is one essential step in the process but it is not the only essential one. We also need to move beyond the negative to embrace the positive. And, ultimately, the most positive experiences we have come from our loving relationships. It is the moments of love that offer us a path to transcending our pain.

What is love? There are, no doubt, a variety of different concepts that may already be familiar to you. These widely accepted ideas are being put in question by a leading force in positive psychology. In her latest book, *Love 2.0,* Barbara Fredrickson asks us to entertain a new and radical departure from what we've come to believe about love. Her challenge is:

"To absorb what the new science of love has to offer, you'll need to step back from 'love' as you may know it. Forget about the love that you typically hear on the radio, the one that's centered on desire and yearns for touch from a new squeeze. Set aside the take on love your family might have offered you, one that requires that you love your relatives unconditionally, regardless of whether their actions disturb you, or their aloofness leaves you cold. I'm even asking you to set aside your view of love as a special bond or relationship, be it your spouse, partner, or soul mate. And if you've come to view love as a commitment, promise or pledge, through marriage or any other loyalty ritual, prepare for an about-face...

Love is not sexual desire or the blood ties of kinship. Nor is it a special bond or commitment. Sure enough, love is closely related to each of these important concepts. Yet none, I will argue, capture the true meaning of love as your body experiences it."[55]

---

[55] Fredrickson, Barbara L. Ph.D., *Love 2.0: Creating Happiness and Health in Moments of Connection,* Penguin Books, New York, 2013, p. 5.

So what is this radical new idea that Dr. Fredrickson is espousing? Simply put: "Love is that micro-moment of warmth and connection you share with another living being."[56] The examples she gives are:

"As you check out of the grocery store, you share a laugh with the cashier about the face you see peering up at you from the uncommonly gnarly tomato in your basket.

On the way to pick up your mail, you happen upon a neighbor you've not seen in a while and pause to chat. Within minutes you find yourselves swapping lively stories with each other about the fascinations you share.

At work, you and your teammates celebrate a shared triumph with hugs and high fives.

On your morning jog, you smile and nod to greet fellow runners and silently wish them a good day.

You share a long embrace with a family member after a trip that has kept you apart for too many days."[57]

The love she describes above is neither exclusive, lasting, nor unconditional as we may have expected based on our ideas of love in the past. Yet it is nonetheless profoundly important to us. As Fredrickson explains:

"Love, it turns out, nourishes your body the way the right balance of sunlight, nutrient-rich soil, and water nourishes plants and allows them to flourish. The more you experience it, the more you open up and grow, becoming wiser and more attuned, more resilient and effective, happier and healthier. You grow spiritually as well, better able to see, feel, and appreciate the deep interconnections that inexplicably tie you to others, that embed you in the grand fabric of life."[58]

For our purposes, it is the arena of health and sickness we are particularly interested in. According to Fredrickson, the

[56] *Ibid.*, p. 10.

[57] *Ibid.*, p. 15.

[58] *Ibid.*, p. 4.

initial step you need to take is to use your own suffering as a bridge to connection.

"Whenever pain, suffering or any form of adversity weaves its way into your own experience, take that very moment as a cue to practice compassion, to take tender care of yourself."[59]

This is equivalent to our first step of "being on your own side." Then, she suggests, you take a step back from your own suffering and imagine yourself connected with others who suffer as you do. This is a movement from self-compassion toward compassion for others and the recognition that you are not alone.

Rising to this level of compassion for self and others begins to break down the walls of isolation that are characteristic of the pain experience. It equips us to be caring and loving to ourselves, to open to the caring and loving we are receiving from others, and at the same time, to learn to be caring and loving to others as well. All three transformations are happening at the same time.

In the end, what I believe is most healing for all forms of sickness and pain is to feel compassion for yourself as you suffer and compassion from and for others who are caring for you. And since "compassion *is* love,"[60] we must conclude that it is the experience of love that helps us rise above pain.

A Peak Experience: Rachel's story

How can you describe a peak experience? It is just the kind of experience where words fall short. Hence it is necessary before we say anything at all, to make it clear that whatever we

---

[59] *Ibid.,* p. 143.
[60] *Ibid.,* p. 142.

end up saying will be more like a glimpse than an accurate description. Words cannot convey the full impact of such an experience.

As you know, my son and I spent sixteen days - or significant parts of those days - together in the hospital. I've also shared some details of how we spent that time - walking the halls (and once, flying down them,) lying side by side in bed watching movies, dining on the patio and, later, sitting at the same table in the dark talking. Sometimes he just sat with me as a calm quiet presence and let me have my bad times. At other times, he lifted my spirits until I could touch my own courage again. He listened to me worry obsessively for ridiculously long periods of time. Then, when I could finally stop fretting to listen, we would figure out a plan of what to do. We were a team. He kept reminding me that we would get through this together - because "we are a team," he would say.

There were so many issues to go through each and every day in hospital, even though, on the surface, it may have looked like nothing was happening. Somehow the time got filled up with more and more details. There were some too embarrassing to talk about since an assault on dignity is a constant in hospital life. There were some medically difficult decisions to wrestle with and resolve. Food was a perpetual topic of conversation, regardless of whether I was off or on it. Why I didn't eat or what I did occupied an inordinate amount of attention. Always - it goes without saying - there was the matter of managing the pain and managing the illness at the same time. Sometimes the hospital itself drove us crazy with its plethora of tests and procedures and administrative demands. We had to be constantly conscious of balancing our time alone and our time together in

*order to honor both our needs. Neither of us had antici-
pated or prepared for such an endlessly long stay. Then,
while all this was going on, there were visitors coming
and going, people calling, Kieran needing our help.*

*It was a remarkably intense shared reality taken out of
and foreign to our ordinary and normal lives. We don't
usually spend time together in anything remotely like
this way. And, as a finishing touch, it was punctuated
every four days by the CT scan rollercoaster of mounting
hopefulness, the agonizing waiting, followed by the
descent into disappointment. This whole complex and
challenging experience was weaving a texture of intense
involvement, intimacy and cooperation that was set
against a background of our shared history – literally,
since my son was born.*

*Then one evening the room lit up and we were infused
with a new radiant energy. Our hearts opened and we
felt ourselves lifted to a new level of love. Pain disappeared. I simply did not notice it anymore. The room was
honey-yellow and glowing. I had learned in Diamond
Heart Training[61] that this was the color and taste of love.
It may sound hokey but when you experience it, it is
unmistakable. People who came in the room felt it. We
were all smiling. It was beautific. I locked it in.*

This was a peak experience. Does it continue like that all
the time? No, sadly, Fredrickson is right; it doesn't last. But the
memory lies in waiting and I can go there to revisit it any time
I wish. At the moment, as I think back on it, my chest expands
and it aches in a wonderful way. I can feel it and it makes me
smile again.

---

[61] Diamond Heart training is a spiritual education based on the work of A.H. Almaas
that I participated in as a student for about three years in the Pacific Northwest and
another two years in Santa Barbara, 1994 to 1999.

People may have peak experiences like this with their partners. I know I did with my ex. In that case, it had a quality of passion that was absent in the experience with my son. I imagine it colored with a sparks of firey red. This may be why people hang on to relationships even when they just aren't working, because a peak experience brings with it a high that is not easily forgotten. My ex used to say: "If God made anything better, He kept it for Himself." Perhaps this is what mystics and saints experience when they connect with God in a kind of spiritual ecstasy that lifts them out of themselves. Such experiences are memorable and transformative. They take us to a higher level. They lift us out of our pain.

Contrary to Fredrickson, however, I would not find such peak experiences of love comparable to laughing with the cashier in a grocery store about a tomato or celebrating a victory with coworkers or greeting fellow runners on your morning jog and silently wishing them a good day. Even a hug with a family member you have missed may not qualify as comparable. I think these examples are on a distinctly different level from the peak experiences I am talking about. They belong in our category 2 of "focusing on the positive." They counter-balance the negative impact of suffering by allowing in an experience of positivity. In this way, they *reduce* the experience of pain. They do not *transcend* it altogether.

Fredrickson does admit: "It's far easier to connect with another person when your desire, bond, commitment, or trust is present and strong."[62] And it seems evident that a positive experience with a person who means something to you as opposed to a total stranger is generally not only easier to attain but also has a different valence. It carries more weight. As a result, it may come to occupy a significantly more impactful place in your mind in contradistinction to the pain you feel at that time. And this counts. It is offering an even

---

[62] *Ibid.*, p. 9.

higher level of relief from pain than the momentary connections with strangers.

However, the peak experience is in a class by itself. It not only reduces the level of our pain; it allows us to rise above pain altogether. When we are infused with a heightened love of this sort, we are able to rise to a level where there is no pain. We are caught up in the exhilaration of being flooded with love. Whether that love is personal or universal, whether with another human being or with whatever we experience as God, it is the pathway to a higher state of being, a blissful state of joy and peace.

I would argue that the bedrock of shared history, an intimate caring relationship and a sense of devotion is not accidental but *essential* to the experience of transformative love. Not just the micro-moments of connection in general but the deep connection that is felt with a person of importance in your life raises us up to this higher level. It is part and parcel of what makes a transformation of this sort possible.

Admittedly, a peak experience is not an everyday event. It is a relatively rare occurrence. Perhaps this rarity is what makes it so intrinsically special that it is able to vanquish our pain entirely, if only for a little while. Yet we must recognize that if it occurs, it is most often in the context of a committed relationship, one where there is a devotion to caring for each other in sickness and in health. Compassionate caring is what paves the way.

Conclusion

By way of conclusion, we will take a brief walk through the book highlighting some of the vital learnings we hope have been received.

In Part One, we saw that being immersed in extreme pain due to an illness or an accident is more than just an experience of physical discomfort. It ushers a person into a whole new world, one that has changed in a pervasive and profound way. The things you will be focused on now are radically different from those things that occupied your mind before this turn of events. In our phenomenology of the pain experience, we traced the aspects of change across a myriad of dimensions affecting your experience of the world, your experience of yourself and others, your experience of time, and your confrontation with the meaning of your life.

If you are a person in pain, hopefully you will resonate with the picture we paint. Perhaps you will feel seen and understood on the deepest possible level. And if you are caring for someone in pain, perhaps it will open the doors to a deeper understanding of the challenges they face in coping with a life of pain on a day to day basis.

In Voices of Pain, we meet a series of remarkable people who offer their personal stories of being flung into a world of pain through illness or injury. If you suffer as they do, they will remind you that you are not alone. What they teach is their lived truth. And for all of us, they bear witness to the amazing power of the human spirit to meet and deal with suffering.

Marilyn tells us about how she learned to curtail her tendency to do for others at the expense of her own well-being. She has developed a new level of appreciation for and sensitivity to her body. Pete explains how he virtually loses a third of his life to migraine headaches. Nonetheless, he expresses gratitude for the other two-thirds of his life that are unaffected. Nancy was an ardent athlete before her leukemia, as was Wendy before her fall from her horse. Both women faced the need to make huge adjustments in their activities and, consequently, in their sense of self. Michael's career as a naval pilot came to an abrupt halt when his back surgery failed to heal his pain, as did Rick's work as a carpenter following his forty-foot fall from a roof. Both men had to reinvent their work lives to adapt to their new limitations and changed abilities. Pat's experience with back pain, although brief, brought her life to a standstill. Previously independent, she became, for a time, completely dependent on her mother to take care of her. Louise suffered extreme pain for months on end from an undiagnosed ectopic pregnancy that rendered her incapable of functioning until, finally, her condition was identified. For the first time, she became aware that her normally unexpressive husband really loved her. Otis suffered two major illnesses involving a series of five surgeries and he credits his wife and her constant support with getting him through this long ordeal. We hear from Justin how a brain tumor diagnosed at the tender age of four had a dramatic effect on the life he lived from that point on. What sustained him through the many hardships of his life were his love relationships. David lives a limited life due to his crushed ankle but has achieved a new appreciation of his Self and, in this process, has woken up to the crucial importance of his family. He goes so far as to say: "I know that this statement will sound strange, but if I could wave a magic wand and make my pain go away, I would not."[63] Then he adds: "How we humans hold the pain we experience, defines us." [64]

---

[63] Cf. above, p.91.

[64] *Ibid.*

The way these individuals hold the pain they experience is inspirational.

In Part Two, we address aspects of the caregiver style such as their energy and quality of touch that may be invisible but nonetheless have a powerful impact on patient healing. We look at the issue of whether and how information is shared with the patient. Are we simply passive followers or involved team members in relation to our medical practitioners? The hospital as the primary place we go to heal is examined in terms of how it, on the one hand, promotes health and, on the other hand, mitigates against health and healing. Two different examples of devastating negative impact are offered as instructive warnings about how the hospital system operates when it is at its worst. Then we turn to focus on the treatment of patients with so-called "psychosomatic" illnesses whose physical symptoms are defined in psychiatric terms. This exposé continues the theme of abuse by the medical system that, we argue, needs to be identified and fought against. It represents a call to action directed toward the medical experts who hold the power to heal or destroy us.

Perhaps as caregivers, you may pause and ask yourself if you can make use of messages in this section to deepen your connection to your patients. Perhaps as consumers, you may find yourself better prepared to avoid pitfalls in the medical system and to promote the best possible level of treatment. And, just perhaps, if patients and caregivers join forces to work together, we can move closer to the ideal model of care that feeds body, mind and soul.

Part Three is a call to action for patients. It reaches out to those who suffer and are searching for answers. How can we reduce, relieve or eliminate our pain? A number of strategies are reviewed and evaluated as roadmaps for pain management and/or recovery, ranging from meditation to hypnosis, from releasing the negative to focusing on the positive. We examine

EMDR as a way of reprocessing painful memories. We look at religious affiliations and spiritual experience as resources to turn to. We consider the constructive role of passionate interests such as art, music, and sports. We explore insights from positive psychology and brain physiology. We illuminate the importance of love in moments of connection as well as in enduring and committed relationships. Finally we turn to peak experiences of love as the ultimate path to transcending pain.

In all these ways, help is possible. The quality of our lives can be improved. We can find moments of joy and a sense of meaning. We are not merely prisoners of a body in pain.

We end on a message of hope. *About Pain* charts the choppy seas of the pain experience with an unremitting honesty about its negative aspects. However, we arrive at a message of optimism. Pain tests us, it stretches us, but in the end, it need not defeat us. We are beings who can, after all, rise above pain.

A Final Word

We started this book with the acknowledgement that most of us recoil from pain, our own and other people's. We don't want to see it or hear about it. But, if you have read the book this far, then you have overcome your initial reluctance and let yourself approach what you could have chosen to avoid. You have walked the path of understanding what millions of us who suffer pain experience on a daily basis. A subject hidden in the shadows has begun to emerge into the light.

As you have delved deeper and come to see pain in its many facets, as you have read stories from people who are bravely reaching out to share their experience of pain, and as you have learned to appreciate the subtle ups and downs of caring for those in pain, it is possible that you have been drawn in the direction of compassion – moving to connect with, not distance, from those in pain. If so, this book has served its purpose. For all of us who suffer and all of us who care, I sincerely hope that it is so.

May I, together with all who suffer, find peace.[65]

---

[65] Fredrickson, Barbara L., Ph.D., *Love 2.0,* p. 144.

About the Author

Dr. Rachel B. Aarons began her professional career as a philosopher. She was awarded numerous scholarships and fellowships including the prestigious Woodrow Wilson Fellowship, the Horace B. Rackham Graduate Prize Fellowship, and the Canada Council Dissertation Fellowship. She completed her Doctorate in Philosophy at the University of Michigan in 1971 and taught at the University of Toronto as a Lecturer and Assistant Professor of Philosophy from 1968 to 1973.

At this point, her career took a new direction. She received a Master's degree in Clinical Social Work from the University of Toronto and also completed a three year training program as a Gestalt therapist at the Gestalt Institute of Toronto. She maintained a private practice in Toronto until she moved to Vancouver, British Columbia in 1978. She was also trained by Virginia Satir as a conjoint family therapist and later became a faculty member of the Northwest Satir Institute.

In Vancouver, Dr. Aarons founded and coordinated a Women's Resource Center and then served as a career counselor for Capilano University before she returned to private practice in Counseling and Hypnotherapy in 1984.

In 1996 Dr. Aarons moved to Santa Barbara, California and was licensed as a Clinical Social Worker for the State of California (LCS 18298) in 1997. She was first trained in EMDR therapy in 1998 and became certified as an EMDR therapist in 2004. She continued her practice as a therapist first under the auspice of the Family Therapy Institute of Santa Barbara for ten years and then in her own private practice. She specializes in helping people move out of stuck places with destructive behavior patterns and negative thoughts using the rapid processing of EMDR therapy.

In 2009, she published *Journey to Home: Quintessential Therapy and Beyond* outlining her theory of the essentials of effective psychotherapy. In 2011, she published her second book, *Therapy at Lightning Speed: Case Studies of EMDR* documenting her work with a variety of different clinical issues.

For the past forty years, Dr. Rachel Aarons has been a companion and guide to individuals and couples on their journeys to growth and healing.

Contact Information:
Dr. Rachel B. Aarons LCSW
1018 Garden Street, Suite 106,
Santa Barbara, CA 93101
Tel. (805) 450-6365
Fax: (805) 617-1700
Email: rbaarons@yahoo.com
www.RachelAarons.com

Bibliography

Aarons, Rachel B. MSW, Ph.D. *Journey to Home: Quintessential Therapy and Beyond,* Journey Press, Santa Barbara, California, 2009.

Aarons, Rachel B. MSW, Ph.D. *Therapy at Lightning Speed: Case Studies of EMDR,* Journey Press, Santa Barbara, California, 2011.

Brach, Tara. *Deliberate Practice and Inner Transformation,* Psychotherapy Networker webinar, December 2014.

Buber, Martin. *I and Thou,* Charles Scribner's Sons, New York, 1958.

Charcot, Jean Martin. *Clinical Medicine and Research,* Kumar et al., http//ncbi.nih.gov/pmc/articles /PMC3064755

Ellenberger, Henri. *The Discovery of the Unconscious: The History and Evolution of Dynamic Psychiatry,* Basic Books, New York, 1981.

Epilepsia, Vol. 44, Supplement 6, International League Against Epilepsy, Blackwell Publishing, 2003.

Felletti, Vincent J. M.D. *The Relationship of Adverse Childhood Experience to Adult Health: Turning Gold into Lead,* Kaiser Permanente Medical Care Program, San Diego, California, 2002.

Fredrickson, Barbara L. and Levenson R. *"Positive Emotions Speed Recovery from the Cardiovascular Sequelae of Negative Emotions,* Psychology Press, 1998.

Fredrickson, Barbara L. *"The Role of Positive Emotions in Positive Psychology,"* American Psychologist, 2001.

Fredrickson Barbara L. et al. *"The Undoing Effect of Positive Emotions,"* Motivation and Emotion, 2000.

Fredrickson, Barbara L., Ph.D. *Love 2.0: Creating Happiness and Health in Moments of Connection,* Penguin Group, New York, 2013.

Hanson, Rick, Ph.D. *Buddha's Brain: The Practical Neuroscience of Happiness, Love and Wisdom,* New Harbinger Publications, Inc., Oakland, California, 2009.

Hanson, Rick, Ph.D. *Hardwiring Happiness: The New Brain Science of Contentment, Calm and Confidence,* Harmony Books, New York, 2013.

Hanson, Rick, Ph.D. *Brain Science and Psychotherapy: What's the Next Step?* Psychotherapy Networker Symposium, Keynote Address, 2014.

Kradin, Richard L. *Pathologies of the Mind/Body Interface: Exploring the Curious Domain of the Psychosomatic Disorders,* Routledge, New York, 2013.

Scarry, Elaine. *The Body in Pain: The Making and Unmaking of the World,* Oxford University Press, New York, 1985.

Simon, Richard. *Reaching into Life: An Interview with Virginia Satir,* PsychotherapyNetworker.org/free-reports/, November 2014.

Spitz, René. *The First Year of Life,* International Universities Press, New York, 1965.

Szasz, Thomas. *The Manufacture of Madness: A Comparative Study of the Inquisition and the Mental Health Movement,* Harper and Row, New York, 1970.

Van der Kolk, Bessel M.D., *The Body Keeps the Score: Brain, Mind and Body in the Healing of Trauma,* Viking by the Penguin Group, New York, 2014.

Voices from the Shadows, https//vimeo.com/on demand.

Weiss, J.S. and Wagner S.H. *What Explains the Negative Consequences of Adverse Childhood Experiences on Adult Health?* American Journal of Preventative Medicine, 1998.

www.ingramcontent.com/pod-product-compliance
Lightning Source LLC
Chambersburg PA
CBHW032100080426
42733CB00006B/355